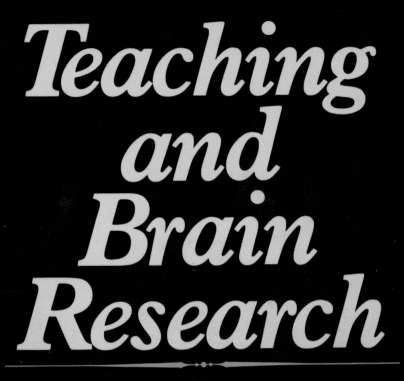

Teaching and Brain Research

Guidelines for the Classroom

Michael P. Grady

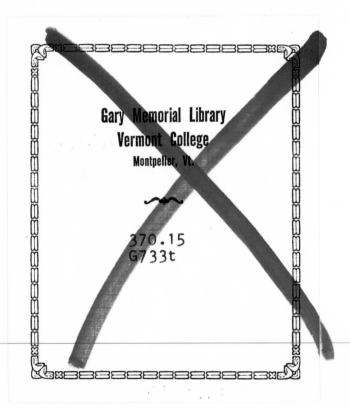

Teaching and Brain Research

Teaching and Brain Research

Guidelines for the Classroom

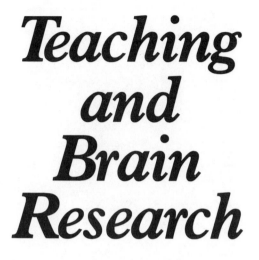

Michael P. Grady

Saint Louis University

Longman
New York & London

For Emily

Teaching and Brain Research
Guidelines for the Classroom

Longman Inc., 1560 Broadway, New York, N.Y. 10036
Associated companies, branches, and representatives
throughout the world.

Developmental Editor: Lane Akers
Editorial and Design Supervisor: Ferne Y. Kawahara
Composition: ComCom
Printing and Binding: Haddon Craftsmen

Library of Congress Cataloging in Publication Data
Grady, Michael P.
   Teaching and brain research.
   Bibliography: p.
   Includes index.
   1. Brain—Localization of functions. 2. Cerebral
dominance. 3. Learning—Physiological aspects.
4. Curriculum planning. I. Title.
QP385.G73 1984   370.15   83-19938
ISBN 0-582-28377-9

Manufactured in the United States of America
Printing: 9 8 7 6 5 4 3 2 1   Year: 92 91 90 89 88 87 86 85 84

Table of Contents

Preface

We are on the frontier of a new understanding about learning and teaching; we are beginning to understand the functioning of the human brain. The emergence of this knowledge will stimulate tremendous advances in educational practices. At last, we will know how we learn and remember and consequently, the most effective techniques for teaching children. This advance will mark the beginning of a new era for educators.

In this book, which is based on ten years of studying brain research and working with teachers on the subject, I have attempted to relate some current thinking on the brain's functioning. In addition, I have developed educational applications, based on brain studies, which are relevant to classroom teaching. These applications are an effort to answer the question most often asked of me: What are the implications of current brain studies for the regular classroom teacher? Obviously, the suggestions in this book are based only on our current knowledge about the brain. This is a beginning, not a complete answer. It is my sincere hope, though, that this book will stimulate educators to study the reports of neuroscientists, make classroom applications, and contribute to the understanding of the brain. Only with this concerted effort of all involved groups will we someday reveal the mysteries of the brain.

I want to acknowledge the assistance of many people in the preparation of this book. Jackie Vernon helped with the initial design and contributed to the classroom applications. Emily Luecke Grady made suggestions about the manuscript and contributed to chapter seven. Caroline Cosentino wrote many of the classroom activities for chapter six. Moreover, many students and teachers provided thoughts from their experience and asked stimulating questions that helped clarify my thoughts. Jack Muhlenbruch provided extensive editing suggestions. Finally, I would like to thank Phi Delta Kappa for their permission to use material from my 1978 PDK publication, *Education and the Brain.*

CHAPTER ONE

Education and the Brain

The brain is the most complex and intriguing part of the human body. It is mystifying that at a time when computers and other complex machines are becoming common items in many homes, we know very little about the brain and even spend relatively little time studying it or applying research findings to the educational process.

Certainly it is appropriate for educators to consider the research of neuroscientists and apply the research findings of these scientists to education. Anyone who has an interest in the brain and related research need not apologize for such interest. The study of the brain is multidisciplinary, requiring many professional groups, including educators, to employ their expertise and unique perspectives in exploring the functions and potential of the brain. This concerted effort will someday reveal the answers to many of today's questions regarding the brain and thus increase tremendously our understanding of the teaching–learning process.

There are various concepts of how the brain functions. None of them is completely satisfactory. Some even contradict one another. This is just one indication of our limited knowledge on the subject. Much more research is needed. The following is based chiefly on what we have learned from research during the past twenty years.

The Hemispheres of the Brain

Research efforts suggest that the brain consists of two hemispheres. While these hemispheres may appear to be similar, there is evidence that they specialize in different functions. The left hemisphere specializes in linear and sequential operations, whereas the right hemisphere specializes in simultaneous and visual functions. (These functions are explained in chapter four.) This finding has considerable implications for curriculum and instruction such as the proper balance of curriculum and instructional strategies that take hemispheric specialization into consideration. The subject of teaching and learning style or, in more general terms, cognitive style, is related to the question of hemispheric organization.

Evidence that the left hemisphere of the brain is primarily linear–sequential and the right is mainly simultaneous–visual raises the question of dominance. Is someone mostly left-hemisphere dominant or right-hemisphere dominant? To help you understand the dimensions of hemisphericity and dominance, consider the following questions:

When traveling to a new place, do you prefer verbal directions or a map?

Do you prefer reading directions for the model you are about to assemble, or can you see how it goes together without the directions?

Do you prefer solving problems intuitively or logically?

Are you good at remembering faces?

Do you prefer working on one project at a time or many simultaneously?

Are you comfortable with ambiguity, or do you prefer precise systems?

Your answers to questions like these may reveal your preference for ways of thinking associated with left-hemisphere functions or right-hemisphere functions.

Here is another example:

In the following puzzle using letters of the alphabet, should the letter G be placed above or below the line?

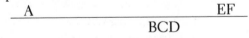

In trying to solve this puzzle, did you begin by thinking numerically: 1 - 3 - 3, or . . . ? Did you look first for a sequential pattern? Through schooling, most of us have been conditioned to look ini-

Through schooling, most of us have been conditioned to look initially for sequential patterns even though they may be inappropriate responses. Perhaps now you see that the solution is in the *shape* of the letters: G goes below the line because it has a rounded shape, not the straight lines found in the letters above the line. Determining the proper shape provided the correct answer, not the numerical sequence.

These examples help to explain what is meant by left- and right-hemispheric dominance when we speak about the functions of the brain. Perhaps you are beginning to understand your personal dominance. Do you prefer linear, sequential, and verbal functions rather than holistic, simultaneous, and visual cues? Or does it make any difference? The answers to these questions help you understand your preference. In addition, your answers can show you how your preference relates to your learning and teaching styles.

As you proceed through this book, you will be encouraged to think about brain research and its implications for teaching and learning. You will also be asked to diagnose your thinking–teaching styles and learn how to expand and balance your teaching in relation to instructional techniques, curriculum, and the brain dominance of your students. You will be urged to use both left-hemisphere (linear) and right-hemisphere (holistic) thinking in solving educational problems.

Using This Book

We wrote this book for elementary- and secondary-school teachers, administrators, and specialists. The first section presents background information from current brain research which will give you some understanding of how the brain functions. The second section of the book contains applications of the hemispheric theory to classroom methods and curricula. You will find a selection of useful activities for many content areas and various grade levels along with explanations and a justification for these approaches in the teaching–learning process. The last section suggests ways for administrators to develop schoolwide programs based on brain-related research, and some possible outcomes of future research from the neurosciences.

This book was written to introduce the results of brain research to educators in order for you to begin thinking about relevant classroom applications. We hope that it serves this purpose and leads you to future discoveries and improved instructional effectiveness.

CHAPTER TWO

Past and Present Findings in Brain Research

At one time there was much prejudice against brain research because most scientists believed that it was impossible for the brain to study and understand itself. But in recent years, as people saw the need for such research, neuroscientists began to explore what may be the most difficult and complex scientific challenge of all time. While brain research continues, many wait for potential rewards such as reducing or eliminating mental illness, solving learning problems, and understanding how children learn and remember.

Former Beliefs

Through the ages there has been a fascination with the brain. Scholars and philosophers of different civilizations have expressed their theories regarding the location of the mind in the body: whether, for example, it is located in the liver or the heart. Now we are exploring the brain in order to understand the mind.

Several "sciences" developed as a result of efforts to explain the brain. Physiognomy, although not dealing directly with the brain, was the "science" of determining personality on the basis of facial and head characteristics. It became popular in the eighteenth century through the writings of a man named John Lavater. His writings made statements such as this: A low forehead and a thick neck indicate stupidity, whereas a high forehead indicates intelligence.

More directly related to brain research was the "science" of phrenology, which described a person's character from the shape of the head. Developed by a man named Franz Gall (1758–1828), this theory claimed that mental qualities were associated with physical characteristics. In phrenology, various parts of the brain are thought of as locations for certain qualities and functions, a concept based on Gall's contention that persons with certain "bumps" on their heads (as described by him) had certain qualities (which he also described) Gall observed the heads of students and thought that he could feel the "organ" of number in mathematicians, the organ of tune in musicians, and so forth. He also thought that a certain bump gave poets their skill and that other bumps made people thieves or murderers.

Today we believe that Gall's theory is false. Because of the protective skull, we can't even tell the shape of the brain by touching the head. There is no evidence to support Gall's claim that the functions of the mind (love, hope, knowledge) are located in specific parts of the brain.

Current research does not support either physiognomy or phrenology. Nevertheless, it is not for us to ridicule these pseudosciences, but to remember that what is being claimed about the brain today may be as inaccurate as phrenology or physiognomy.

Current Explorations

Once scientists overcame the prejudice that it was impossible for the brain to understand itself, tremendous advances were made. Many of these advances became possible as a result of technological innovations such as brain-wave measurements, sophisticated x-rays, and chemical analyses. These inventions have been extremely helpful in studying the brain.

Along with these technological advances, a new field of study has emerged: psychobiology. This field incorporates brain research and the behavioral sciences. It differs from other fields of study that attempt to understand behavior because it starts with what we know about the brain and how it functions. In general, psychobiology deals with the mind's effort to know itself through the study of the brain. It attempts to answer, on the basis of brain research, questions that were previously discussed by philosophers and theologians: What is reality? How do we know? What is truth? Efforts to answer these questions will ultimately assist us in understanding behavior as we interact with students in school settings.

The following paragraphs summarize some interesting concepts about the brain as revealed through recent research.

Plasticity

An important finding is that the brain has what is called plasticity; that is, it has an enormous capacity to reorganize itself. Although it does not regenerate new brain cells, it can form new connections among existing neurons. This organization of new connections takes place at all ages, but it is greatest in children up to the age of twelve, when it levels off. The brain is so plastic in the young that children who lose up to one-half of the brain can grow up to have normal intelligence. It is during these early years that most children learn so much, including language, usually with little effort. (We tend to ignore this fact when we persist in teaching foreign languages only at the high-school and college levels.)

What does this research mean for the educator? It suggests that experience, as well as the basic mental makeup with which the child enters the world, can greatly influence and shape the brain development of the child. If experience shapes the functioning of our brain, then the educator needs to determine when it is appropriate to teach certain subjects, which instructional techniques are most effective, and in general, what can be done to develop children fully.

Brain Waves

Experiments have been conducted in the use of brain-wave readings to develop a foolproof lie-detector test, determine how we think, or explore how we make decisions. Brain-wave tests have also been used to measure intelligence or diagnose mental and physical abnormalities. Through proper diagnosis, it is possible to suggest methods for the remediation of difficulties brought about by abnormalities.

One example of how tests of brain-wave function can help educators is the detection of dyslexia in children of preschool age. If this disability can be determined early enough in the child's life, remedial or other appropriate programs can be initiated at once rather than waiting for a diagnosis that may come too late to help the child effectively.

Sex Differences

Recent evidence suggests that the brains of the two sexes may have different physical and chemical characteristics. At one time, it was thought that differences in male and female interests were determined socially. But now it appears that males and females may be predisposed toward different talents from birth, and that this is due to brain differences. Apparently societies have reinforced and increased these differences throughout history.

The difference between male and female shows up in the organization of the two hemispheres of the brain. For example, women are thought to be superior in verbal abilities whereas men are thought to be superior in spatial abilities. Women tend to be more bihemispheric (can use both hemispheres appropriately) than men. Continued experiments regarding sex-related differences support the theory that such differences do exist.

What are the educational implications of sex differences? Perhaps we need to look at the makeup of the average elementary classroom. Is the classroom structured in a way that enhances the learning of girls and inhibits the learning of boys? If it is true that boys prefer manipulative and visual activities, perhaps elementary classrooms are creating learning-disabled and/or hyperactive boys. Why are certain disciplines (engineering, physics) dominated by men? Could it be due to the way these subjects are taught in the classroom? Do we need to examine teaching methods in order to incorporate learning activities involving functions of both hemispheres of the brain? Why are foreign-language programs dominated by women? It appears that differences in brain functions between the sexes do exist. As we search for more answers to our questions, it appears that we should take a closer look at sex differences in relation to brain functioning and schooling.

The Chemistry of the Brain

Dr. Avram Goldstein pioneered research efforts leading to the discovery of beta endorphins and enkephalins, potent brain chemicals, a discovery that may change our understanding about mental illnesses, learning, pain, pleasure control, and other areas of mystery surrounding the brain. Experimentation and experience indicate that the brain employs some kind of method for differentiating between pain and pleasure, and between that which one wishes to remember and that which is not remembered. With better understanding of the chemistry of the brain, it will be possible to change the functioning of the brain through the use of drugs similar to natural brain chemicals. This area of research is thought to be particularly promising for the thousands of people who suffer from mental illness.

By providing new ways to explore and explain the functions of the brain, Goldstein's discovery adds important data to previous findings. For example, we have gained further understanding of the well-known "placebo effect." Placebos or sugar pills are chemically inert substances used to lead patients to think that they are receiving a particular medication when in fact they are not. After taking a placebo, many patients report an improvement such as a lessening of pain. Why patients report relief when they have not actually received any medication has puzzled scientists for years. It now appears that people who have received placebos report relief because, for some reason or other, there has been an increase in the endorphin level. This finding suggests that the brain has the power to make physiological changes by itself as well as when it receives external chemical stimulation. Through endorphin research scientists may be able to invent medicatons that are not addictive or do not have harmful side effects. Indeed, endorphin research may reveal the secrets of the chemical basis of behavior, a finding of immense importance to educators.

Other Areas of Development

The following are other areas of brain research of interest to educators:

Artificial eyes for the blind. Using a miniature television camera to transmit impulses to the brain may allow blind people to see.
Artificial ears for the deaf. A device that bypasses the damaged

sensory system will bring impulses directly to the hearing center of the brain.

Foods that may enhance our ability to learn and remember. Researchers are experimenting with chemicals to improve learning and modify behavior.

Even though we have learned much about the brain that will be helpful to educators, we have solved only a fraction of the brain's mysteries. The eventual answers to the questions of how we learn and remember and whether we are using our brains correctly will have far-reaching effects on the educational process and increase tremendously the effectiveness of teachers and schools. As researchers find additional answers to questions about the functioning of the brain, educators will surely find this information exciting and helpful.

New Considerations

One should note that increased knowledge about the brain brings new considerations and cautions. We do not simply have the power to increase learning. We also have the power to control the mental development of others. In time, it appears, we will know how to program the brain to do or think as we believe it should. Scientists who know how the brain works will have the potential to control the minds of others. Indeed, sophisticated brainwashing will truly be a reality. Further, accurate mind reading may become a very real possibility.

While it is exciting to realize that in coming years our understanding of the brain will increase dramatically, we realize that developments will raise new ethical and moral questions, some of the most important ever to confront mankind. Who, for example, will control our minds? Who will have authority to read our minds? Who will determine what is good for us? These ethical issues may well be the next level of brain research after the brain understands itself.

CHAPTER THREE

How Your Brain Works

It is beyond the scope of this book to provide lengthy details regarding the functions of the brain. *The Brain: The Last Frontier,* by Richard M. Restak, is a comprehensive book on brain research. Restak suggests that one way to understand the operations of the brain is to consider three major components: *alertness, information processing,* and *action.* The interaction of these three units is required for the brain to function. To sit quietly looking out a window, for example, requires the interplay of all three brain elements.

Scanning movements of the eyes are taking place all the time as we look for essential clues about what's going on in front of us. At the same time, we are registering and synthesizing sights and sounds which enable us to realize, for instance, that we are looking out on a playground. If we observe a toddler fall off a swing, the combined action of all three functioning brain units will result in our hurrying out to comfort him. Trying to pin down what part of the brain is involved in the perception of the child's fall is like trying to describe the precise location and movement of a subatomic particle. (Restak, p. 44)

Within the approximately three pounds of matter we call the brain lie these complex functions of alertness, information processing, and action. The brain also contains an electrical system that can be traced on an electroencephalogram and a chemical system composed of neurotransmitter chemicals that either transmit or block the electrical impulses. It is a system more complex than the most sophisticated computer. The brain is simultaneously conscious of its existence and adaptable to it. In this small, soft, grayish lump of tissue are generated dreams, feelings, and learning.

In this chapter we will examine some concepts of how the brain functions. First, however, we will discuss the question of the brain and its relation to the mind.

Brain/Mind

Can we use the two terms *brain* and *mind* interchangeably or is there a significant difference? The traditional answer to the brain/mind question has been that the mind represents the action or functioning of the brain. Previously, the mind was a meaningless concept unless discussed in terms of the brain. Today we realize that the brain/mind question is more complex than we thought. Some researchers suggest that it is more appropriate to think about the brain as a process rather than a three-pound lump of matter. The brain is required for the mind, but it would be incorrect to equate the two in a cause–effect relationship because we would be attempting to relate two different processes. In other words, it is insufficient to use the term *brain* in explaining the workings of the mind; the brain is important in understanding the mind, but it is not the simple cause of why the mind functions. The processes of the mind are much more complex and follow their own patterns of existence. The mind is dependent on the brain, but at the same time the brain is dependent on the mind. The historical argument regarding brain/mind continues.

What, then, is the relationship between the brain and the mind, and how do we distinguish one from the other? Although this problem may never be solved, we are achieving more satisfying perspectives on it by thinking of the brain as a process rather than as a thing. Karl Pribram, whose model of the brain we examine next, presents one interpretation of how the brain functions as a process.

Holographic Memory

Karl Pribram, a noted neuropsychologist, uses a model based on holography to explain how the brain distributes and stores information. Holography is a method of lensless photography that uses a laser light's single frequency to construct holograms (patterns or pictures). The laser light strikes the object and impinges on a photographic plate at the same time as a reference beam (light from the same laser but reflected from a mirror) arrives at the film. Because the two waves have the same frequency but strike the plate at different angles, their interaction forms an interference pattern which is recorded on the plate. The plate appears as a meaningless pattern of swirls but any part of the hologram will reconstruct the entire image. When the hologram is placed in a laser beam, the original wave pattern is regenerated and a three-dimensional image appears. If the hologram is successful, it is difficult to tell the projected image from the real.

How does this rather complex phenomenon relate to brain function? Pribram suggests that brain information storage may be like a hologram in that the brain distributes information across an entire surface. Memory seems to be distributed throughout the brain rather than being localized in a particular part. Since information is stored in the brain like images on a holographic plate, any section of the brain can recreate the entire memory. This theory may explain the puzzle of why, even when 50 percent of the brain is destroyed, an individual still retains most of his memory and does not remember only half of his acquaintances. There is no direct correspondence between how much tissue is damaged and how much memory is lost.

The "brain hologram" is one concept developed to explain memory. (Only a brief description has been presented here. Further reading is encouraged.) It is hoped that through the discovery of dynamic patterns of the biological holograms in the brain, some parts of the brain's functioning will be understood. If the theory proves accurate, it may provide the model of how sensory input is distributed in the brain, stored as memory, and later reconstructed. The theory may also provide an answer to the question, "How does the brain know?" and assist educators in their attempt to improve the teaching–learning process.

Brain Development in Terms of Growth Spurts

Mental development is linked to and limited by the development of the brain. The neurosciences have recently given us data that suggest a new way of looking at educational strategies, curriculum, and evaluation. This data is the basis for the theory of growth spurts during brain development, espoused by Herman T. Epstein.

The formation of brain cells ceases early in life, probably before the end of the second year. The cessation contrasts markedly with the increase of about 35 percent in brain weight after that age. This increase of brain weight suggests an increase in the complexity of neural networks in the brain. If this increase in the complexity of neural networks occurs continuously, then the development of a child at any age represents a point on a continuum. On the other hand, if increases in brain weight are not continuous, but rather occur at discrete periods, then we need to think in terms of stages of brain development which may be correlated to stages of mental development.

Epstein has suggested that human brain growth occurs "primarily during the age intervals of three to ten months and from two to four, six to eight, ten to twelve or thirteen, and fourteen to sixteen or seventeen years, and that these stages correlate well in timing with stages found in mental growth" (*Education and the Brain*, eds. Chall & Mirsky, p. 344). He also points out that development during the age period of ten to twelve is slightly earlier for girls and slightly later for boys. This situation is reversed in the fourteen to sixteen brain growth period.

Given the body of facts we have sketched regarding brain development, one can think of possible implications for learning in general and for schooling in particular. One working hypothesis would be that intensive and novel intellectual activities for children may be most effective during the stages of brain growth. Anatomical data might be interpreted to infer that novel challenges presented at a time when the child's mind is not prepared to receive them might cause an active and potentially permanent turn-off of the ability to absorb some of these challenges at a later and more appropriate age. While it is tempting to propose further hypotheses at this point, the question of what to do during the "fallow" periods can be answered definitively only by conducting in schools some well-designed experiments focused directly on that question.

One can think of some additional possible implications based on the brain growth-spurt theory. Stemming from the previous description of spurt and fallow periods, new light may be shed on the problems of junior high or middle schools. Youngsters in these schools are usually ages twelve to fourteen, a fallow or plateau period of brain development, according to Epstein. Perhaps we are over-challenging students at this age by insisting that they make mental leaps for which they are not ready. Educators may need to rethink the development and requirements of students between twelve and fourteen. The correlation between current school practice and brain development may be inappropriate.

A similar situation exists in the fallow period of ages four to six. This is traditionally the time when we begin teaching children to read. This timing suggests that we need to reexamine reading readiness, how children can be taught by other methods than reading, and what an appropriate curriculum for the child between four and six would be.

Although these and other inferences can be drawn from this research, it is too early to make decisive conclusions about curricula and instructional strategies. We still do not know how to determine when a child's brain growth is beginning or ending or exactly where growth occurs in the brain during spurt periods. Answers to these questions will aid us further in designing appropriate curricula and instruction for specific students in order to challenge them intellectually at the correct age.

The Triune Brain

"In its evolution the human forebrain has expanded to a great size while retaining the basic features of three formations that reflect our ancestral relationship to reptiles, early mammals and recent mammals . . . a triune brain" (*Education and the Brain,* eds. Chall and Mirsky, p. 308). Thus wrote Paul MacLean in referring to what he called "a hierarchy of three brains in one," a primal mind, an emotional mind, and a rational mind. The primal and emotional minds can't read or write, he said, but still we must deal with them educationally.

The Reptilian-like Brain and the Primal Mind

Observations of reptiles reveal that they are slaves to routine, precedent, and ritual. Such conformity has survival value. We are aware of our own propensity for routine. It becomes such an important part of our lives that we become upset when the routine is broken. Perhaps it is the reptilian brain which at times still causes us to act in primitive ways, as in committing crimes.

The Paleomammalian Brain and the Emotional Mind

In the evolutionary line from mammal-like reptiles to mammals, the young are cared for rather than eaten. Psychologically, this development amounts to the evolution of a sense of responsibility and what we call conscience. The reptilian brain has only a rudimentary cortex. It is believed that during a period of transition the primitive cortex grew and became further differentiated. The term paleomammalian brain or "old mammalian brain" refers to the activity of the mind that processes information in terms of emotional feelings that guide behavior required for self-preservation and the preservation of the species.

The Neomammalian Brain and the Rational Mind

Since there are indications that insistent signals from the inside of the brain make it difficult for an organism to arrive at the coldly reasoned decisions required for survival, MacLean used the term "neomammalian brain" to indicate the period of development culminating in the human brain as presently perceived. In the neocortex (rational mind) there are nerve cells devoted to the production of symbolic language and the associated functions of reading, writing, and arithmetic. In addition, the new cortex promotes the preservation and procreation of ideas and is necessary for language, speech, and the other ways in which we can express ourselves. While vocalization is of questionable significance in the communication of reptiles, it is of vital significance in mammals.

For some inexplicable reason nature added something to the neocortex which brings a sense of compassion to the world: the prefrontal lobe provides foresight in planning and helps us gain insight into the feelings of others. "It is this new development that makes possible the insight required for the foresight to plan for the needs of others as well as the self. . . ." (MacLean, *Education and the Brain,* p. 340). If it is possible that the neocortex is incapable of coming into full operation until adolescence, then it would be incorrect to claim, as some do, that the personality is fully developed and rigid by the age of five or six or even by the time of adolescence.

The triune concept also raises questions about moral judgments and cultural values. There is evidence to indicate that if neural circuits of the brain do not become operational at certain critical times of development, they may never be capable of functioning. For example, if one raises chimpanzees in darkness, they may never see. One may never develop empathy if it is not experienced at a critical age.

These and other observations are significant with regard to the triune brain because we usually assume that we are dealing with only a single intelligence. Because the two older mentalities lack the power of speech does not mean that we can ignore their intelligence or their influence on schooling and how we learn. We need to look at the implications for the schooling of the triune intelligence consisting of a primal mind, an emotional mind, and a rational mind. When we discover how to look at schooling through these three different mentalities, more mysteries of how we learn will be solved.

Summary

This chapter introduced some of the more significant and generally recognized theories regarding brain function. For obvious reasons it is not a complete encyclopedia of knowledge about the brain. (For additional reading see the resources listed at the end of the book.) It is hoped that the chapter does provide some information about the complexity of brain functioning in addition to some current theories explaining how the brain works. Now we will take a closer look at the hemispheres of the brain.

CHAPTER FOUR

The Brain's Hemispheres

In the previous chapter, we briefly examined several models that were developed to explain the functioning of the brain. In the present chapter we will explore what is called the "hemispheric model." We are exploring this model in depth because it is currently considered a very significant model in helping educators understand some of the workings of the brain. The remainder of the book will discuss the implications of hemisphericity for education.

Hemispheric Specialization

Some people have accepted the hemispheric theory as a virtual panacea for the ills of education. Many arbitrary, capricious, and unsubstantial claims have been made about the functions of the two hemispheres. Nevertheless, the data regarding foundational differences between the two hemispheres, now supported by years of research, have significant implications for the teaching–learning process, especially in the areas of curriculum and instruction which we discuss in this book.

A basic understanding of the hemispheric model is necessary in order to understand the educational implications. A. L. Wigan was one of the first to discuss the two hemispheres:

The Mind is essentially dual, like the organs by which it is exercised. . . . The idea has presented itself to me, and I have dwelt on it for more than a quarter of a century, without being able to find a single valid or even plausible objection. . . . I believe myself then able to prove 1. That each cerebrum is a distinct and perfect whole as an organ of thought. 2. That a separate and distinct process of thinking or ratiocination may be carried on in each cerebrum simultaneously. (*The Duality of the Mind*, 1844)

For centuries researchers from many disciplines have speculated about the mind and the brain. References to the apparent dualism of the mind or the two halves of the brain appear in the writings of John Dewey, Thomas Aquinas, Fyodor Dostoyevsky, Arnold Toynbee, and others. The hemispheres became important in the field of medicine in the 1960s when Roger Sperry carried on his experiments with epileptics, work for which he received the 1981 Nobel prize in medicine. Today hemispheric research is extremely fashionable. Journals are replete with reports of various experiments conducted from many points of view.

Early Experiments

Roger Sperry and Joseph E. Bogen gave detailed reports regarding their efforts to alleviate uncontrollable seizures in epileptic patients. After observing that traditional means of treating these patients had failed, Bogen severed the corpus callosum, the nerve fibers that connect the two hemispheres of the brain. For most patients, following surgery, the seizures were less severe and the patients could be treated by using ordinary epileptic medication.

Experiments with patients whose corpus callosum had been severed provided the data on which the distinction between the functions of the two hemispheres is based. Roger Sperry speculated that in these patients each half-field of vision had its own visual images and memories. Through visual tests he determined that what is observed in one visual field (hemisphere) is seen and remembered separately from what is observed by the other visual field. This difference also appears in speech and writing. Visuals, which for most right-handed people are projected to the left hemisphere, can be described through speech and writing. When the visuals are projected to the right hemisphere (through the left visual field) the subject will say that he did not see anything. But if you ask this same patient to use his left hand to select from a group of pictures one that he just saw, he can point to it even though he just denied seeing anything. Other fascinating experiments by Sperry and his colleagues produced essentially the same results. It appears that dividing the brain surgically also divided the brain into two different modes of consciousness.

Hemispheric Organization

In many ways, Sperry's and his colleagues' finding was just the beginning of much research on the hemispheres of the brain. These researchers determined that the two halves of the cerebrum, while seemingly alike, have unique characteristics. The right hemisphere controls the motor and sensory operations of the left side of the body, the left hand, and half of each retina of the eyes. The left hemisphere controls the same operations on the right side of the body. The corpus callosum connects the two hemispheres and integrates their operations. In addition, each hemisphere specializes in a particular mode of consciousness. On the basis of experiments with patients who had their corpus callosum severed (described previously), and also on the basis of experiments with patients who suffered brain damage, researchers have hypothesized that a person has two ways of processing stimuli and that each seems to stem from a separate hemisphere.

Instead of the normally unified single stream of consciousness these patients behave in many ways as if they have two independent streams of conscious awareness, one in each hemisphere, each of which is cut off from and out of contact with the mental experiences of the other. In other words, each hemisphere seems to have its own separate and private sensations; its own perceptions; its own concepts; and its own impulses to act, with related volitional, cognitive, and learning experiences. (Roger W. Sperry, "Hemispheric Disconnection and Unity in Conscious Awareness," *American Psychologist*, 1968, 23, p. 724)

The left hemisphere specializes in linear, sequential, and analytic operations whereas the right hemisphere specializes in simultaneous, holistic, and metaphoric operations (see diagram). Based on research results, educators are currently speculating that each hemisphere specializes in a different cognitive mode. This specialization and

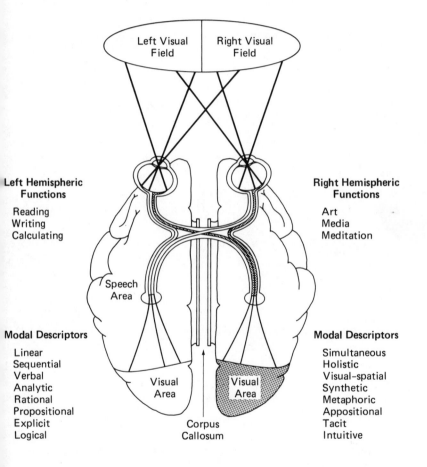

Left Visual Field

Right Visual Field

Left Hemispheric Functions

Reading
Writing
Calculating

Speech Area

Modal Descriptors

Linear
Sequential
Verbal
Analytic
Rational
Propositional
Explicit
Logical

Visual Area

Right Hemispheric Functions

Art
Media
Meditation

Modal Descriptors

Simultaneous
Holistic
Visual-spatial
Synthetic
Metaphoric
Appositional
Tacit
Intuitive

Visual Area

Corpus Callosum

interrelatedness may be of specific help for educators in understanding teaching and learning processes.

Modes of Consciousness

The two dominant modes of consciousness are the right-hemispheric (simultaneous) and the left-hemispheric (linear) processing systems. Functions of the two modes are activities associated with one or the other of the two. For example, reading, writing, and arithmetic are among the functions of the left-hemispheric mode which utilize the linear–sequential processing system. Art, visual media, and metaphor are functions of the holistic right-hemispheric mode of consciousness. In most individuals there seems to be a hemispheric preference for specific functions. At times a function can be lateralized in the opposite hemisphere or even show mixed dominance. For example, language may use metaphor, as is seen in poetry, and there may be many sequential elements in spatial perception. Although the language function may lateralize primarily in the left hemisphere, it is not exclusively left hemispheric, as we know from the experiences of people in Eastern cultures (where some languages lateralize in the right hemisphere) and people whose left hemisphere has been damaged; in these cases, the right hemisphere has taken over the language function. Once information enters the brain, both hemispheres can work cooperatively to process it. Specialization in the hemispheres does occur, however, in the modes of consciousness if not always for particular functions.

Learning Styles

The discovery of the two dominant modes of consciousness leads educators to a discussion of preferred learning styles. The question arises: Do students have a preferred method of learning? To put it another way, do students learn more effectively through verbal, linear, analytical, and logical processes or through visual–spatial, metaphoric, and holistic processes? If a student has a preferred mode of learning or cognitive style, how does the teacher determine this and how does he or she use this knowledge in teaching? Another question is: How do we utilize the functions of both hemispheres of the brain in the teaching–learning process? These and other questions that have to do with hemispheric specialization will be addressed in succeeding chapters.

Handedness

Handedness, the tendency to use one hand rather than another, relates to hemispheric specialization. Left-handers, about ten percent of the population, have often been ridiculed because of their handedness. We know many stories about youngsters who were forced to write with their right hands even though they preferred the left. If you look at the meanings of the words—"sinister" means left in Latin, "right" means correct—you see more prejudice. (This distinction also holds in some other languages.) When a student gives a correct answer, you never say, "That's left"; you say, "That's right." Other prejudices certainly exist, but at this point we want to look at the relationship between handedness and hemispheric specialization.

What "causes" a person to prefer the use of one hand over the other? Various explanations for left-handedness have been presented. They include the claim that hand preference is learned, that left-handedness is caused by some birth trauma which presumably damaged a part of the brain controlling right-handedness, and that left-handedness is caused merely by a recessive gene. These theories have the appeal of simplicity but lack support from research results.

Whatever the cause of hand preference, many researchers believe preference reflects the fact that the brain functions asymmetrically, despite its apparent structural symmetry. In other words, some of the brain's functions are laterally differentiated between hemispheres. As stated earlier, the left hemisphere is believed to be superior to the right when sequential, logical stimuli are presented, and the right is believed to be superior when dealing with visual or configurational aspects of stimuli. These differences have been assumed to underlie contrasting cognitive styles. At one time, it was thought that left-handers were the converse of right-handers in terms of hemispheric specialization. (The left–right functions were lateralized in opposite hemispheres.) Recent studies indicate, however, that most left-handers, like right-handers, have their verbal functions lateralized in the left hemisphere.

Although a single theory to identify and explain a handedness and cerebral specialization relationship has not yet been established, at least three variables that affect results have been identified: sex, degree or strength of handedness, and family history of (left-)handedness. Females show less hemispheric differentiation of functions than do males. It is not known why this is so. When degree of handedness is considered (right-, left-, or mixed), the degree of lateralization differs. Whether subjects have left-handed relatives also affects results. It is not clear how these variables interact, but they affect the degree of lateralization. Whether being left-handed improves or hinders a student's ability to succeed in school and in specific subjects is also unclear.

In general, the evidence suggests that when the family history of handedness is considered, two distinct groups of right-handers and left-handers emerge. In the group of left-handers with one or more left-handed relatives (and only in this group) bilateral speech and visual functions occur. This is a very small percentage of students. On the basis of hand preference alone, left-handers' cerebral organization cannot be reliably distinguished from their right-handed counterparts. Perhaps future research studies will give us more information about handedness and in particular about the characteristics of left-handers and how to teach them most effectively.

Summary

Through hemispheric research, we have gained some understanding, or learned in a new way (one with a physiological basis), about the manner in which people think. Perhaps, because of methods in and out of school which stress left-hemisphere dominance, we are dominantly linear–sequential thinkers. This situation may be adequate when a problem is solved best through linear–sequential processes, but when a problem requires holistic and simultaneous processes, it is possible that we will arrive at an incorrect solution. It seems that an over-reliance on left-hemisphere thinking, in which we have been grounded, has caused us some unnecessary problems. If, through hemispheric research, we place more emphasis and value on right-hemispheric skills, we may improve our ability to solve problems and be able to help those students whose cognitive style is holistic, simultaneous, and visual. We are learning to diagnose the thinking styles of people, often through unobtrusive measures. As we learn more about diagnosis, we will learn more about how people think and how they are likely to learn best. This knowledge will be of immeasurable help to teachers.

CHAPTER FIVE

Applications of Hemispheric Specialization

In many classrooms, the teaching–learning methodology is based primarily on the linear, sequential, and analytic functions of the left hemisphere of the brain. An examination of the curriculum of many schools also shows that the curriculum is often weighted with subjects that stress the linear–sequential mode of reasoning. Subjects such as reading, writing, and arithmetic employ linear–sequential processes heavily. It appears, however, that equal emphasis should be given to methods and subjects which employ the simultaneous and visual functions of the right hemisphere. The integration of these two sets of hemispheric functions (linear–sequential and visual–simultaneous) will help balance instruction, increase learning, and provide effective instructional techniques for more students.

The Unbalanced Curriculum

What does the traditional curriculum require of students? Both elementary and secondary students are usually given verbal directions to complete a linear task. Most instruction involves "teacher talk" while students listen. This style often overlooks students who learn in other ways, such as visually or kinesthetically.

In other classrooms, learners are asked to read assigned material and then write answers in response to written directions. Students who experience difficulty in reading usually find it difficult to express themselves in writing. The student should have the option of responding to questions in one of a number of different ways, including oral or pictorial responses.

In the study of mathematics, students are often assigned a series of equations to compute. Although math is a linear subject, it also involves visual thinking in the computational process and in higher logic. For this reason simple computation should often be presented in graphic form. Visual logic needs to be developed in addition to verbal and written logic.

The back-to-basics movement which stresses reading, writing, and arithmetic is likely to ensure that in many schools learning activities that depend on functions of the left hemisphere will continue to be emphasized over those that depend on the right hemisphere. Generally a teacher is pleased if students perform correctly all the tasks relating to the basics: the teacher may even describe such students as superior, working to the best of their abilities. In reality these students are using only half of their potential, half of their thinking abilities, half of their brains; they are neglecting the other half.

Balancing the Curriculum

Various balances should be considered when constructing a curriculum. As a result of his study of hemispheric specialization and current curricular trends, the author suggests that a school curriculum should be examined in relation to left–right specialization and integration. It is not my intent to remake or destroy the present curriculum, but to bring about more integrated approaches to teaching and learning. A balanced curriculum is one that stimulates both hemispheres through the use of the multiple processing systems of the brain.

In an article in the *UCLA Educator* entitled, "Some Educational Aspects of Hemispheric Specialization" (Spring 1975), Joseph E. Bogen suggests that the brain's right hemisphere receives little, if any, organized, deliberate schooling. The balanced curriculum suggested here can be implemented through interdisciplinary approaches. Adding subjects to the curriculum is not necessary. To some extent art, music, movement, and creative thinking already exist within the school structure. Hemispheric research has served as a catalyst for the development of interdisciplinary studies in which teaching and learning can cross content lines. An integration and blending of areas such as reading and music, and art and science: require both right- and left-hemisphere processing as students find new forms of creative expression. Even though the value of the interdisciplinary approach has been recognized by educators for years, teaching and learning have generally stressed those activities requiring specialization in left-hemispheric functions.

It is important to look at the present curriculum to determine whether it is unbalanced. The following questions may prove helpful to teachers, administrators, and students alike:

1. How much emphasis is there on basic subjects that stress left-hemisphere thinking?
2. If the subjects taught are left-hemisphere oriented, are they taught in a way that uses both hemispheres of the brain?
3. Does the curriculum provide for an integrated approach to learning in which the teaching and learning process cuts across content lines?
4. Do the subjects allow for productive–creative thinking that makes it possible for students to express their understanding in a variety of ways?
5. Does the testing program provide for qualitative evaluation strategies?

Student Evaluation

Just as the school curriculum may be out of balance in the sense that it places too much emphasis on left-hemisphere functioning, school evaluation procedures, too, draw heavily on left-hemisphere functions. Much evaluation, both teacher-developed and standardized, focuses on the student's ability to deal with linear and sequential functions. Most tests measure the ability to understand in written terms and require students to answer in writing. Rarely does one find tests that use visual language rather than verbal to measure understanding. It is likely that many students are being misjudged because of their inability to use written forms to express their understanding and knowledge.

Current grading practices are inadequate in that they are grounded in linear recording, involving letter grades, percentages, and numbers (which constitute a linear scale of achievement). These sequential orders, honor rolls, and deans' lists encourage competition and comparison. Very few schools use qualitative evaluation measures such as interview, observation, or creative evaluation techniques.

Evaluation is an area where the holistic approach can benefit all students, whatever the subject or teaching–learning situation. Creative evaluation that allows students to express themselves in ways other than paper-and-pencil tests can expand the potential for productive thinking and creative problem solving.

Getting Started

Teachers may feel incapable of changing the curriculum in their schools. If so, the author advocates that teachers use the freedom they have within subject areas to include teaching strategies, materials, and evaluation techniques which require the use of the functions of both hemispheres of the brain. The teacher who is truly concerned with integrated learning can overcome the curricular restrictions.

In reaching students, it is important to involve as many senses as possible so that each individual learner has an opportunity to perceive knowledge through his or her preferred learning style. Left-brain dominant students and teachers prefer teaching–learning situations based on authority and written forms. Right-hemispheric dominant students and teachers process information best when it is presented in a visual, tactile, or kinesthetic mode. They need to see pictorial examples, have material explained in visual terms, and have the opportunity to manipulate materials.

Teachers need to determine the preferred mode of learning, for themselves and for each student. This determination can usually be done through simple observations such as whether a student is an avid reader and writer but dislikes gym class, or whether a pupil can take apart a bicycle in five minutes but shows no interest in mathematics. Given a choice, most students and teachers use their most comfortable mode of learning.

Observation and Evaluation Instruments

There are a number of tools, such as the "Learning Style Inventory" developed by Rita and Kenneth Dunn and Gary Price, which assist both students and teachers in determining their preferred learning styles. The Learning Style Inventory (LSI) is a useful tool in analyzing the conditions under which students prefer to learn. These conditions include: a. immediate environment (sound, heat, light and design), b. emotional climate (motivation, responsibility, persistence, and structure), c. sociological needs, (self-orientation, peer orientation, adult orientation, or combined ways); and d. physical needs (perceptual preference(s), time of day, food intake, and mobility).

The LSI asks questions to determine how students learn. For example:

I study best when it is quiet.

I have to be reminded often to do something.

I really like to mold things with my hands.

I do better if I know my work is going to be checked.

I study best at a table or desk.

The things I remember best are the things I read.

I try to finish what I start.

I can ignore most sound when I study.

I like to study by myself.

I really like to draw, color or trace things.

The inventory summarizes the students' responses which can be used to identify an individual's learning preferences and achieve maximum individual academic progress.

Another instrument, "Your Style of Learning and Thinking Test," developed by Paul Torrance, at the University of Georgia in 1976, sheds light on individual problem solving and thinking styles.

Questions such as the following assist in determining whether a student is right-hemisphere or left-hemisphere dominant or has integrated problem-solving and thinking styles:

a. I respond best to verbal instructions.
b. I respond best to instruction by example.
c. I am equally responsive to verbal instruction and instruction by example.

a. I prefer multiple choice tests.
b. I prefer essay tests.
c. I have equal preference for multiple choice and essay tests.

a. I prefer classes where I have one assignment at a time.
b. I prefer classes where I am studying or working on many things at once.
c. I have equal preference for the above type of classes.

If after observing a student the teacher wishes to identify the individual's preferred mode of learning, these instruments may be helpful. Identification of learning styles has been a practice in special education for some years: why not in other educational settings?

Children need not be labeled as having only one learning–thinking style. They will receive a better education when the teacher balances instructional strategies to reach as many senses as possible. In the process, each student can learn through his or her preferred mode and at the same time gain access to knowledge in a variety of ways. As a result, the individual develops both modes of thinking and uses the whole brain in a manner similar to the way a pianist uses both hands—one playing the main theme while the other plays the accompaniment to create the final product.

Balancing Instructional Strategies

Using balanced instructional strategies is a way to reach an entire class of students in a situation where individualized instruction is impossible. The following are ways to stimulate individual children and their learning styles while still meeting the needs of the entire class during the presentation of new or review material.

1. Through observation and a keen awareness of students as individuals as well as members of the group, make an assessment of each individual's preferred mode of thinking.

2. Introduce material in a variety of ways, giving both verbal and visual directions. Allow students to take notes and also read the written material from a text. Provide opportunities for students to manipulate materials and to observe demonstrations.

Each content area has the capacity to be presented in several ways, thereby enriching the body of content and making not only learning but teaching more dynamic and interesting. Teachers should welcome the opportunity to present their material in verbal and visual–spatial terms, and also welcome student participation and interaction. Role playing, overhead transparencies, maps, charts, and manipulative objects can help learners visualize and verbalize their responses to content.

3. Occasionally the teacher should present material in only one mode or emphasize one learning–teaching style. This allows students to stretch their thinking and problem-solving abilities, and to react to material in a style different from their preferred mode of learning. Individual students may be assigned specific work to challenge them to think in ways other than their preferred learning style.

At times material can be presented solely through verbal instruction, challenging students to be attentive listeners. When this is the procedure, students should receive only verbal directions for a task and then respond verbally with their answers. At other times, material can be presented only in written form, requiring students to read carefully for meaningful concepts. Written directions, followed by written responses, awaken students to the literacy involved in the reading and writing of content material.

A sound–slide or video tape show with accompanying material can stress visual images and visual stimulation. Students may be asked to give a pictorial or graphic response, giving them the opportunity to expand the visual–spatial mode of thinking.

A Classroom Example

The following is a description of a classroom where the teacher accepts the challenge to present material in a variety of ways, thus allowing students to practice their preferred mode of thinking and expand their capacity to include a variety of senses. The teacher's objective is to provide integrated instruction and learning.

Mrs. Macy is a seventh-grade science teacher in a medium-size middle school located in a rural community. Science is required for all students. Her classes are large. The lab tables are placed around the perimeter of the room rather than in rows, making it possible for students to focus their attention on a large demonstration table in the center. Mrs. Macy often uses an overhead projector during her discussion of scientific concepts. She supplements her teaching with slides, tapes, filmstrips, and transparencies, many of which are made by her and her students. She has organized an article and pamphlet file in which she and the students collect items of interest on science, ecology, and space exploration. The room is visually exciting and colorful. Vegetable plants are growing near the windows. Charts and graphs enliven the walls. Students use science units as themes for bulletin-board displays. Bookshelves are used to display student projects and experiments.

Mrs. Macy prides herself on her ability to present science material in a variety of ways. She explains each concept verbally, visually, and graphically. She assigns a wealth of supplementary reading material. She still gives tests in written form, of course, but often she asks students to respond to her questions verbally or debate a point of view, in order to test their comprehension of an entire concept or body of knowledge. Several students tape their verbal answers to test questions. Mrs. Macy listens to these verbal answers and grades them the same as those that are written. (Most students in the class still prefer to give written responses, but at least once a semester she challenges them to verbalize concepts on tape.) Students also have the option to do projects which may include written reports, graphs, charts, or scales that illustrate their experiments and observations. They may give oral reports or construct scale models.

This science teacher does not write separate lesson plans for various presentations and lectures but includes the different modes of presentation in one master plan. She believes that lesson planning and activity development should center around the content of the curriculum according to the age level of students. The content determined by the school curriculum should be the basis for teaching but can and should be presented in a variety of ways and evaluated in a variety of ways.

Sample Lesson Plan
for the Holistic Teaching
of a Science Concept

Lesson Title: The Human Skeletal System; Joints in the Human Body

Objectives: Explain the function of a bone joint in the human skeletal system.

Name two types of joints and the movements they allow.

Identify joints within the human skeletal structure.

Materials: Human skeleton, if available; X-rays from a hospital; diagram of the human skeleton (overhead transparency); diagram of ball-and-socket joints (overhead); straws, string, tape, cardboard, foil.

Modes of Presentation:

Verbal: Explain concepts verbally, stressing important vocabulary words.

Visual: Use overhead transparencies and hospital X-rays. Have students picture concepts visually, stressing important spatial relationships.

Written: Supply students with reading material explaining concepts of joints and their movements. This may be from a textbook or supplemental material.

Manipulative: Give students string, straws, tape, cardboard, and so on. Ask them to construct both types of joints with these materials and explain their construction to the class.

Assignment: Have students identify joints in their own bodies.

List the type and location of each type of joint (i.e., shoulder ball-and-socket; elbow-hinge; hip ball-and-socket).

Activities: Enrichment—Have students reconstruct a chicken skeleton, labeling all the joints. Use this model to continue the study of the skeletal system.

Summary

The individual learning styles of students can be enhanced through a variety of instructional strategies so that the students' knowledge of the content area is more holistic and meaningful. The hemispheric specialization theory supports the inclusion of holistic subjects in the curriculum in addition to instructional methods that employ integrated visual–spatial strategies.

The following guidelines will help teachers develop both visual and verbal thought processes in their students.

1. Encourage students to picture concepts or objects visually before giving verbal answers.
2. Give directions and explanations both visually and verbally in written and manipulative forms. Allow time for experimentation and creative problem solving.
3. When giving assignments, allow students the option of illustrating an idea (with pictures, diagrams, etc.) or expressing themselves in words.
4. Occasionally attempt to stimulate one hemisphere only, thus expanding thinking in the nonpreferred mode.
5. Be aware of each student's preferred mode of learning, whether it be linear or visual.
6. Strive for holistic thinking that encourages the student to use a variety of thinking skills to solve problems and comprehend content.

This last point refers to the most important goal of teaching: integrated thinking. To meet the needs of educators and learners, formal schooling must stress all modes of consciousness.

CHAPTER SIX

Content Area Activities
K–8

Each content area in elementary and secondary school curricula contains a unique body of knowledge, concepts, and skills. These content areas also offer students the opportunity to develop and strengthen right- and left-hemispheric modes of processing specialized information.

The activities in this and the following chapter suggest specific instructional classroom strategies that incorporate both right and left-hemispheric functions. The activities involve the left hemisphere's capacity to organize, sequence, analyze, reason and verbalize, they also incorporate the right hemisphere's capacity to process information holistically, visually, intuitively and simultaneously.

Many of the activities have been field-tested successfully. The results have been positive and thought provoking. Students learn if given the opportunity to process information in their preferred mode, but they are also challenged by the chance to broaden their experience in the use of the nonpreferred mode of learning. By stressing both right and left brain processes, more integrated thinking and learning are achieved.

These activities are a starting point, a way for teachers in all fields to begin to look at content from a holistic and integrated point of view. We emphasize that this is only a beginning, not a panacea. Problems may arise in the implementation of these and other activities related to brain research, but an understanding of the brain's functioning will, in the end, produce more effective teachers and increased achievement.

The activities are grouped according to subject: Social Studies, Science, Mathematics, Language Arts, and Multidisciplinary activities.

Social Studies Activities

A WORLD APART

Grades 3–4

This is a graphic method of demonstrating to youngsters the concept of the hemispheres of the earth. Using manipulatives assists those students who learn well through tactile methods.

Objective
· To demonstrate the hemispheres of the globe.

Materials:
· Ball of clay (2–3″ circumference), one per student or one for the entire class.
· A wire to cut through clay; pencil for engraving the equator.

Procedure
· Locate the equator by carving it into the ball of clay.
· Locate the north and south (or east and west) poles.

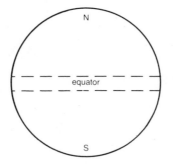

· Refer to a world map to name continents and countries located close to the north and south poles.
· Slice through the ball and separate the two parts in order to

help students understand the concept of the hemispheres of the earth.

Evaluation

- Have students do this exercise themselves. You can then observe their understanding of the hemispheres of the earth.

WORLD MAP: LOCATING MAJOR POINTS OF REFERENCE

Grades 3–4

This is a multimedia activity that is helpful for students learning the concepts of continent versus country and ocean versus sea. The students will also be able to locate major points of reference on a map. This extensive project requires several days in order to include all of the learning modalities used in the activities.

Objectives
- Students will be able to locate on a map the seven continents, five oceans, and the Mediterranean and Caribbean seas.
- Students will be able to name from memory the seven continents, five oceans, and the Mediterranean and Caribbean seas.

Materials
- Globe (more than one, if possible).
- A wall map of the world.
- World map or overhead transparency with only the continents drawn in.
- One map of the world per student with only continents showing.
- If possible, one film on the geographic and cultural characteristics of each continent.
- Crayons and markers.

Procedures
- Explain concepts of continent versus country and ocean versus sea.
- Use overhead transparency or wall map to locate continents, oceans, and seas, describing each in terms of its neighbor, then . . .
- Each student makes a world wall map that includes only the seven continents, five oceans, and two seas, or . . .

- Each student makes a papier mâché globe that includes only the seven continents, five oceans, and two seas. (Additional materials are needed for these last two projects.)

Evaluation
- Based on the assignments:
  –Correct labeling.
  –Relative location, size, and shape of continents and oceans.

MORE ON MAPS

Grades 3–6

After students have been introduced to a specific geographic area through a film, and have been further introduced to elevation maps and raised relief maps, you may proceed with this activity. This exercise allows students to explain their understanding of maps through visual and graphic processes.

Objectives
- To interpret an elevation map.
- To create a raised relief map.

Materials
- Flour.
- Salt.
- Water. (Use sufficient amounts of all three to make a dough mixture, enough for the whole group.)
- Bowl.
- Cardboard or posterboard sheet, 12″ × 18″.
- Pencil and eraser.
- Film of geographic area under consideration.
- Elevation map (of considered area).
- Poster paint (colors relative to key of elevation map).
- Paint brush.
- Newspaper.
- Paper towel, hand towel, rag.
- Space for drying the maps.

Procedure
- Students need first to draw the elevation map on their cardboard (just the outline is needed). When they are satisfied with their map, they need to decide how high the highest areas will be, and from that judge the height of the other areas. If there are areas

below sea level, their system will have to show that. The dough can be mixed after the outline of the map is drawn.

- The dough should be spread to make the raised elevation. Allow one day for drying.
- When the maps have dried, students may paint them according to the colors on the map legend. If anything needs to be written, a permanent marker is best because it affords greater control than paint.

Evaluation

- The students' understanding of relief maps is determined by the overall quality of the project, especially their attention to detail.

CHARACTER PRESENTATIONS

Grades 5–9

Character presentations cause students to analyze research material to discover the character of the person they will play. The students then must synthesize the material into a characterization. Further, the students integrate their learning into a presentation which they perform.

Objectives
- To gather information from three to five sources about a Black American.
- To use the information to develop a characterization of that person for an interview.
- To give a convincing character presentation of a famous Black American.

Materials
- Reference material, nonfiction books, and biographies of persons selected by students.
- Videotape equipment, if available.

Procedures
- Students can work alone or in groups.
- Students choose one Black American they are interested in and research his or her family background, childhood, education, personal struggle, goals, values, humorous stories, accomplishments, and so on.
- Students should be able to complete the interview form that follows this section.
- Students may then practice with each other for their performance of "An Evening with _____" (their character's name).
- The show will follow a "talk show" format, with the host or hostess interviewing the famous character using the interview list for a guideline.

Interview Questions:

  Interview sheet for _____ (name of guest) _____

1. Date of birth and death _____
2. Age at time of interview _____
3. Important historical events during lifetime _____
4. Family background (parents, spouse, children, brothers, sisters, where you lived, who you lived with, and so on) _____
5. Significant events during childhood _____
6. Education ___ _____
7. Favorite story about your family or childhood _____
8. Important influences on your life _____
9. Accomplishments _____
10. For what are you most famous? _____
11. What led to this accomplishment? _____
12. Any other interesting/funny information _____

Evaluation

· Evaluate the students on their knowledge of the Black American, their preparation, their synthesis of the material, and their overall performance.

STATES ON PARADE

Grades 2–4

This activity combines art and history. Students research a state's major contribution and then design a shoe-box float to show off that contribution. Verbal and visual processes of the brain are combined in a task that all students can accomplish.

Materials
- A variety of art supplies are needed. Or, the students may be able to make the float at home.

Procedure
- Students may work alone or in pairs.
- Students need to gather some background information about a state and consider what major contribution it has made to the United States.
- Students will then design a float using a shoe box.
- The float demonstrates that state's major contribution.
- Have students brainstorm how they might represent the state's major contribution.

Alternative
- This same concept can be used to represent nations.

Evaluation
- A group of teachers can judge the floats and awards can be given.

Science Activities

DISCOVERING THE DIGESTIVE SYSTEM

Grades 3–6

This project-oriented exercise provides insight into the digestive system. Building a lesson around a project provides for a variety of learning styles and thought processes. Students who may not do well on a paper-and-pencil test may perform well on this kind of activity, which allows for more visual and holistic thought processes.

Objectives

- Students will name the parts of the digestive system.
- Students can describe the functions of given parts of the body.
- Students will develop a concise visual description of the digestive system.

Materials

- A film on the digestive system.
- A model of the human body.
- An overhead transparency or a poster of the digestive system.

Procedures

- Teacher provides instruction or material on digestive system.
- Students' project is to represent the information on the digestive system in a visual story form.
- Several formats can be used, depending on availability of equipment: videotape, film, slide–tape shows, large picture book.

Evaluation

- The students' projects can be judged by a group of teachers, and awards can be given.

HEALTH TIPS

Grades 4–7

This activity combines verbal and visual functions in the production of a public service announcement for television. The PSA promotes health care.

Objective

- To summarize an important health-care principle in a public service announcement for television.

Materials

- Props may be found or created. Clay or papier mâché may be used for making props. A puppet stage might also be helpful.

Procedure

- Develop a list of concisely stated health rules based on class discussion.
- Working in groups of two or three, students are to develop a short (one minute) commercial that explains one of the health-care principles.

Evaluation

- This exercise could be used as a unit or semester review. The students may be evaluated on their commercial.

MAKE NO BONES ABOUT IT!

Grades 4–6

Some animals can fly, some animals can hang by their tails, others can hop, swim, or fish for their own food. Have your students think about the bone structure of an imaginary animal and what different things the animal might be able to do. How about a Rinofeazebel?

Materials
- Paper and pencil.
- Pictures of animal skeletal systems.

Procedures
- Have students prepare a picture or a model of the skeletal system of an imaginary animal that can perform the activities listed below:
    1. Fly long distances.
    2. Fish for its own food.
    3. Land in water without drowning.
    4. Hang by its teeth.
    5. Run on tiptoe.
- Have students name their animal.
- Have students draw a picture of their animal the way it looks when sitting in front of its own house.
- Have them write a story about why this animal is an endangered species.

Evaluation
- Did the students understand the basic animal skeletal systems and their functions?
- Were the students able to represent their animal in a three-dimensional model or did they prefer a two-dimensional figure?
- Were they able to place logically their animal in a habitat and describe it visually?

- Do the children understand what it means when an animal is an endangered species?
- Were the children able to name their imaginary animal creatively?

MAN OR MACHINE

Grades 5–9

Ask students what happens when they put money into a candy machine. Ask them whether the machine "knows" how much money to return or that they have put in the correct amount. When they press "gum," why don't Lifesavers come out? Given that a machine can make decisions, this activity involves finding out how.

Materials

- Reference material on simple and complex machines.
- Drawing paper.
- Drawing media: pencils, pens, markers, and so on.

Procedures

- Students research the workings of simple and complex machines.
- Open up a candy or coke machine with the help of the vendor and have students explain the working parts.
- Have students draw a scale model of the machine's working parts, showing each function of the machine from the coin slot to the candy in their hands.
- Have them think about more complex machines. Plan visit to a machine shop. Students may learn to take apart a bicycle. Some machines need people to operate them, others do not.
- Have students design their own machines, drawing a scale model on paper or actually using parts to assemble it. What function does it perform?
- Ask students how it will help them make decisions.

Alternatives

- Students often take machines for granted. Show them the complexities and "thoughts" behind the working parts of machines they use every day.

Stress planning and machine design. Scale models help students visualize sequence of events and working parts.

Younger children may want to make imaginary machines and bypass the actual construction.

Evaluation

Did the students gain a better understanding of machines, their functions and uses?

Mathematics Activities

PLACE VALUE AND REGROUPING

Grades: Primary

This activity involves verbal, written, visual, and manipulative processes. Teacher and students discuss questions, solutions, and generalizations. The instructor will use the chalkboard to illustrate students' work and will write the generalizations developed by the students. The students use counters (straws) to solve number problems and to discover more efficient ways of obtaining the solution to the problem than counting the straws one at a time.

Objective
- To discover an easy-to-use grouping pattern for adding large numbers.

Materials
- Counters, such as straws (about fifty per student).
- Rubber bands or fifty five-inch lengths of string for making bundles.
- Chalkboard or overhead projector.
- Paper and pencils.

Procedures
- Begin by giving about fifty straws per every two students.
- Ask students to use the straws to solve problems that you state. For example, 23 plus 16; 34 plus 21.
- After students have counted a great deal, ask them if they can figure out a more efficient way to count.
- Have them try various suggestions to determine what works the best.
- Perhaps someone will recommend grouping by 10s—its advantage is ease of counting.

Alternatives

· Have students bundle most of their straws into 10s, leaving some for units.
· Have students work addition problems using the counters.
· Give students written problems on paper, find answers with counters, write down answers.

Evaluation

· Written assignments.
· Determine whether students are using counters correctly in class.

SUBTRACTION

Grades 2–4

This activity encourages the use of manipulatives for teaching subtraction. Using manipulatives increases learning opportunities and helps integrate the visual and verbal modes of learning.

Objectives

- To perform subtraction with one regrouping, using manipulative regrouping.
- To show that subtraction is done with a finite set.

Materials

- Counters, such as straws. Bundle most in 10s; leave others loose. You must also be able to take the bundles apart and put them back together again.

Procedures

- Have students all work the same problem. Try to use realistic situations where counters represent the items. For example: Leo has 23 cupcakes to bring to school. He eats 7 on the way to school. How many are left?
- Students must first get 23 (two bundles plus three).
- Now students must show how they took out seven.
- Wait for an answer, then unbundle a group of ten and remove seven.
- How many are left? 16.

Alternatives

- Students may either work together or independently.
- Use story problem format on worksheets with students using counters.

Evaluation

In addition to checking for correct answers, determine whether students are unbundling the counters only when regrouping is needed.

ADDITION FACTS

Grades 1–3

Counting materials are used by students to discover and define addition facts. Students will progress form counters to worksheets that have visual representations of counters, and choose correct groupings in order to complete the equations.

Objectives
- Students will select groupings to equal a stated total.
- Students will express groupings as a written equation.

Materials
- Fifty beansticks (or other counting material) with either three or four beans to a stick.
- An overhead projector or chalkboard.

Procedures
- In course of lesson, discuss how students can make seven from

- Students will use beansticks or other grouped counting material to find answers to verbal questions such as: How can you pick up exactly thirteen beans?
- Students will move from counters to worksheets that have visual representations of counters, and choose correct groupings to complete the equations. For example:

$$4 \qquad + \qquad \text{\_\_\_\_} \qquad = 11$$

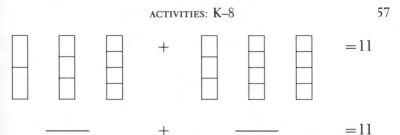

_____   +   _____   =11

Evaluation

You can ask students to demonstrate solutions using counters.
Students can be asked to complete worksheets in window pane,
beanstick, or other grouping styles using the above format.

NATURAL MATH

Grades 4–6

Mathematics, a linear subject, also involves visual thinking in the computational process. Looking at the structural and symmetrical properties of natural objects can be a basis for understanding measurement, balance, and the visual–spatial properties that are so nicely illustrated in nature. Visual and verbal logic are developed.

Materials

- Natural objects such as a bird's nest, an acorn, salt crystals, a soap bubble.
- Metric meter stick.
- Metric scale.
- Formula for the computation of area.
- Pencil, paper, and crayons.
- Camera.

Student Tasks

- What do mathematics, a bird's nest, an acorn, or a soap bubble have in common? Answer these questions and write or illustrate your conclusions.
- How would you compute the approximate area of each object?
- Using metric measurement devices, measure the height, width, or circumference of the object. Put the objects in order from the lightest to the heaviest, smallest to the largest, and so on. What other ways of ordering can you think of?
- Try to draw a scale model of these natural objects using the measurements you have collected. Using your observation skills, look for patterns, lines, and shapes to include in your drawings.

Evaluation

- Did students enjoy working with natural objects or find their own object in nature on which to base their mathematical computations?

Did students use metric measures correctly?

Did students attempt to draw their conclusions instead of writing them or expressing them verbally?

lternatives

Have students find five other natural objects and answer the preceding questions about these objects.

Allow students to photograph other objects that demonstrate symmetry or mathematics in nature.

TEACHING AND BRAIN RESEARCH

RIGHT ANGLES

Grades 4–6

This exercise employs many different modalities of learning in ord
to teach students the concept of right angles. Children can lear
through the functions of both hemispheres of the brain.

Objectives
· To fold paper into a right angle.
· To find examples of right angles in the classroom.
· To compare parts of the body that can be moved to make rig
  angles.

Materials
· A scrap of paper—about 3″ × 5″
· Pencil.
· About five colored circle stickers per student.
· A blank piece of paper.

Student Tasks

A. · Take the piece of paper and fold it in half. Fold it in half aga
     in the opposite direction. What does this part look like?
     corner angle)
   · Put your pencil along one fold. Hold down the end that's
     the corner you've made.
   · Swing the pencil across to the other fold line—it's just gor
     through a right angle. Trace this corner or right angle on th
     other piece of paper.

B. · Now, let's find some right angles around the room. We'll u
     the circle stickers to mark them. Where do you see right angl
     around here?
   · Use the right angles the students made with the paper to prov
     that they are right angles.
   · Get many answers and have the students mark them or yc
     mark them if the students cannot reach them.

- Is there anything we can move so as to form right angles?
- How far would you turn to make a right angle? Get up and try it. How many right angles would you make if you turned halfway around? If you turned completely around? If you turned around twice?
- Now try turning parts of your body to create right angles. Which parts can you move so as to make:
  - One right angle?
  - Two right angles?
  - Three right angles?
  - Four right angles?
- Which parts of your body are most flexible for turning?
- (This activity could be used as a lead-in for the directions and compasses.)

Evaluation

A test could follow this activity on right angles. Perhaps the test could include demonstrations of right angles by the students.

Language Arts Activities

ONE PICTURE IS WORTH A HUNDRED WORDS

Grades 6–12

Someone once said: One picture is worth a thousand words. This activity gives students an opportunity to translate from visual to verbal expression and vice versa.

Materials

- A photograph or painting with some detail.
- Pencils.
- Paper.
- Camera.
- Mounting board (optional).

Procedure

- Have students choose a painting that makes a statement (i.e., crowd scene, landscape, or cityscape).
- Have students study this visual statement and put their visual imagery into writing.
- Limit them to one hundred words (the left brain will appreciate this).
- Students should make their written statements full of description and imagery. Students should make these statements grammatically correct.
- After the writing is complete the students, armed with cameras, should try to recreate or capture the essence of their literary work in a photograph of their own creating (right brain comes through).

Evaluation

The teacher can evaluate both the written and visual work of the students according to agreed upon criteria. Students who don't do well in one area may shine in the other.

A THREE-DIMENSIONAL BOOK REPORT

Grades 6–12

In an effort to use and integrate the thought processes of bot
hemispheres of the brain, try something as simple as changing th
usual method of written composition to create a model or illustra
tion. Both methods (written and three dimensional) can be used t
determine a student's response to a book. In addition, the mode
building and oral explanation give the student who is not skilled i
writing an opportunity to excel.

Objective
- To have students communicate their evaluation of a book in
  nonwritten format.

Materials
- Determined by the students.

Procedure
- Students develop a model or illustration which depicts the them
  of the book.
- They explain their interpretation to the class.

Evaluation
- Students can be evaluated on their model or illustration, the
  interpretation, or on their presentation.

PICTOGRAPHS

Grades 2–6

Combining words and their meanings and the visual representation of the meanings can help students better understand the written word.

Objective

· Students will depict word meanings in creative visual form and use the dictionary to build a vocabulary.

Materials

· Dictionary (Pictionary).
· Drawing paper.
· Drawing media—pencils, pens, markers, and so on.

Procedures

· Expose students to words that have specific meanings and that can also be interpreted pictorially. For example:

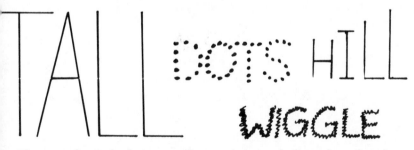

· Have students look up word meanings and then describe the meanings through pictures.
· With younger students, give them simple words to represent, or show them pictographs and have them define the meanings orally.

Evaluation

- Did students create various ways to depict one word?
- Did students increase their vocabulary or discover new word meanings?
- Could children use several pictographs to construct a complete sentence?

CREATE A PHOTO ESSAY

Grades 6–12

Photography is an activity that students as well as adults enjoy. Put photographic creativity and essay writing together, and students can create their own short stories and even books.

Materials
- Any type of camera.
- A subject or theme.
- Plenty of writing paper.
- Mounting board or notebook.

Procedures
- Photo essays can be written in two ways:
    1. Write the story first and take the pictures to accompany the text; or
    2. Take the pictures, sequence them, and write the text to accompany the pictures.
- Have students choose a subject or theme that interests them. They should think the story through and sequence the events of the story, before making an outline of the story sequence and either writing the story or beginning to take the pictures in order.
- After the pictures have been processed, students are to arrange them in order, mount them neatly, and print the text or story under them. The text could be written in prose or poetic form.
- Students can add their own illustrations to complement the theme or let the pictures do all the "talking."
- If the story has characters, the students will need to have other students, adults, or animals pose for their pictures.

Evaluation
- Were students able to plan and pose pictures, being creative in their pictorial representations?

- Did students see the project through from start to finish, ending with a completed product they can be proud of?
- Did students use correct grammar, sentence structure, dialogue, punctuation, and so on in their writing?
- Did students develop or improve photography skills to obtain the effects they wanted to represent?

STORY WRITING

Grades 7–12

This activity uses verbal and visual processes to develop a sound track for a short film. In order to make this task more demanding and interesting, the sound track is for a film that is shown in reverse. This is an intriguing exercise that integrates hemispheric thinking processes.

Objective
- To compose an interesting sound track for a film that is shown backwards.

Materials
- 16mm film, 5–10 minutes in length.
- Tape recorder.
- Recording tape.

Procedure
- Show the film to the class and give instructions for the assignment.
- The class works as a whole to determine the plot.
- Students write the dialogue.
- Students select the background music.
- Dialogue and music are combined and recorded.

Evaluation
- Evaluation is focussed on the sound track, which can be judged by your class or another class.

FIGURES OF SPEECH

Grades 3–6

Figures of speech or metaphors are ways of using language to create pictures. This metaphoric activity can be used in the classroom for teaching literal meanings of figures of speech in addition to creating images through language.

Objectives

- To associate a figure of speech with its literal meaning.
- To play with literal and figurative language.

Procedures

- You will need to list for yourself about fifteen figures of speech and their meanings. For example:

    "She put a bug in his ear to take her out to dinner." (gave a hint)

    "Jane coughed her head off." (coughed a lot)

    "He seems to have a frog in his throat." (unable to talk clearly)
- Write the figures of speech on the board.
- Students are to write and define the figure of speech and then illustrate its literal meaning on the other side of the paper.

Evaluation

- Students can be graded on their correct responses.
- Students can think of different figures of speech or create their own metaphors, using both language and visual art.

RIDDLES, RIDDLES

Grades 4–7

Playing with words can take language out of the linear–sequential sequence and put it in a metaphoric–holistic pattern. Riddles are one way of playing with language. This metaphoric use of language can enhance our power over words and language and engage our right-hemispheric processes.

Objectives
- To list characteristics of riddles.
- To use characteristics of an item to create a riddle that describes the item without naming it.

Procedure
- Begin the activity with an example of a riddle.
- Have students write the riddles in a group first, then write them individually.
- Use riddles to create unusual definitions of words—perhaps the definitions will be remembered more easily by the students.

Evaluation
- Reward students for the most interesting and visual use of words.

Multidisciplinary Activities

PUZZLES AND PROBLEMS

Grades: Varied

Many brainteasers, puzzles, and games that can be used in the classroom are available. These devices employ various learning processes associated with the hemispheres of the brain. They can be fun in addition to providing a method for using various modes of thought in problem-solving situations.

Objectives
- To practice developing alternatives to reach a solution.
- To work in a situation that requires persistence.

Procedures
- There is a variety of material available on problem solving. You can find books that contain puzzles that "bend the brain." In general, puzzles require students to try many possible solutions and to be aware of misleading assumptions. Participation in puzzles can also be used to discuss personal reactions to the problem situation and what techniques are effective in solving puzzles. The following reactions may surface: I was scared; I got mad; I wanted to see what everyone else did; I wanted to quit; I just stared into space.

Tasks
- The following are some examples of typical brain teasers:

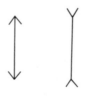

1. Which line is longer? (A science/art lesson could be done on optical illusions.)

```
•   •   •

•   •   •

•   •   •
```

2. Connect the dots using four straight lines. Do not lift your pencil or retrace a line.

3. "Brothers and sisters have I none, This man's father is my father's son." Who is talking here?

- Many other available puzzles assist in developing new ways of thinking. These puzzles can be valuable classroom aids in developing little-used thought processes.

BRAINSTORMING: FINDING SIMILARITIES

Grades 3–12

The following activities are variations on brainstorming. They provide challenges for students to think holistically and to use both hemispheric ways of thinking to develop innovative ideas and solutions.

Objectives

· To develop divergent and alternative thinking.
· To build an accepting, noncritical environment in which students may experiment with the challenges offered them.

Tasks

· Each student is to state one way in which two objects are alike. Agree as a group to stated rules that:
   1. Everyone is expected to give one answer.
   2. The group will wait until each person has given his or her answer.
   3. Do not try to be funny.
   4. Do not comment on anyone's answer.

Materials

· Any two objects may be used.

Procedures

· Seat class in a circle.
· Explain rules as stated in "Tasks."
· Teacher holds up two objects and asks class to tell how they are similar.

Alternatives

· Use a list of words. Ask students to think of ways in which they are alike. For example:

house	hammer	monster
sandwich	water	shoe
chocolate	concrete	hat

- Use a familiar object such as a jug, plastic bag, box, hammer, etc. Ask students what each object could be used for. Move from obvious to more original answers. For this activity, responses could be taken from volunteers to increase the pace. Responses can be listed on paper or a chalkboard.

- This brainstorming procedure can be used to come up with solutions to real problems and may involve the whole class. For example:

    1. You can't find a pencil.

    2. You think that your friend is mad at you because he or she did not talk to you at recess.

    3. You are part of an Indian tribe that lives along a river in an otherwise dry area. The tribe has grown and people are now moving inland as far as three miles from the river. The river has plenty of water. What could be done to provide water for people and crops not immediately along the river?

    4. You are an executive in the car manufacturing industry. Government reports indicate there is a defect in the electrical system that could cause a fire. The company is encouraged to call back the cars and correct the problem. This will cost the company a great deal of money. What are the possible courses of action the company might take?

Evaluation

- Brainstorming responses are usually not evaluated. However, the process can be evaluated based on the quality of the solutions and student participation.

RUNNING A STORE

Grades 6–10

In this activity, students will learn the basic procedures associated with the development of a small retail store. This exercise brings together modes of thinking in a concrete way on a subject with which children have experience.

Objectives
- Students will plan how to operate a small candy store.
- Students will evaluate plans for strengths and weaknesses.
- Students will refine their plans.

Tasks
- To draw a floor plan to scale, including basic furnishings appropriate to the business.
- To provide a list of equipment, merchandise, and other costs associated with opening the business.
- To list potential problems in setting up the physical arrangement of a new business.

Procedures
(Verbal)

- Students will interview or hear a lecture from someone operating a store and be responsible for asking questions.
- Students will be instructed on the basic components to be included in their plan: for example, furnishings, location, rent, utility costs, supply lists, and so on.
- Students will receive verbal feedback on their plans.

(Visual)

- Sample floor plans will be shown.
- Charts can be used for keeping lists and orders, or order blanks from actual businesses may be used.

- A trip to a small business can be arranged.

(Written)—guidelines supplied by teacher

- Resources given for legal requirements.
- A model plan can be given to students in order to establish expectations.

(Manipulative)

- During the field trip, students will see what is needed. Visits to suppliers may be made to compare equipment and merchandise.

Evaluation

- Was the plan for the store developed according to the criteria?

TIME

Grades 4–9

At some point in the year, discussion of future developments—what the future holds—takes place in most classrooms. This activity is an effort to initiate student thinking about the past, present, and future.

Objectives

- To create a time-line of the students' lives which will be used as a reference point for past and future.
- To justify the prediction of the future based on reading and discussion.

Tasks

- Use a long piece of paper (butcher paper, for example) so that students can make a time-line of their own lives. It may appear like this:

		I start preschool.	
1	2	3	4
My first birthday.	My sister is born.	I get my dog, Andy.	We move to Chicago.

I start kindergarten.			
5	6	7	8
I meet my best friend, Joe.	I start piano lessons.	I go on a car trip to New York.	I will go to third grade.

- Students can then be asked to make comparisons on their personal time-lines. This activity can also be extended to include events in United States history which they remember. The time-line can be extended even further to represent world history. The students' time-line would be a point of reference for past events.

- The time-line can also be used to predict the future. Students can create a time-line of the future which indicates when some specific event might take place, or develop their own ideas on future developments, such as:

    When will all cars use synthetic fuel?

    When will the average human lifespan extend to 120 years?

    When will everyday moon travel be available?

    When will teachers program computers to teach rather than teach in person?

    When . . . ?

Evaluation

- You might want to look for justifications for events in the future or details included in the students' time-lines.

ADVERTISING

Grades 5–12

This exercise combines visual and verbal processes in the production of an advertisement. The students can also use brainstorming techniques to develop the new product for which they are going to create an ad. Finally, the students will work together in ad agencies, which requires teamwork and the division of duties.

Objective
- The student teams will develop a convincing ad for a new product.

Materials
- Determined by the students.

Procedures
- Have students divide into groups, giving them all the appropriate cautions about the necessity of having good partners in order to work successfully.
- Discuss advertising methods with the students and show examples.

Tasks
- First, the students must develop a product that their peers do not need, but might be talked into buying. The cost and nature of the product is the responsibility of the students.
- After the students have developed the products, they must produce ads for them. The focus is to convince the target audience that there is a need for the product.

Evaluation
- It might be possible to have an advertising executive judge the results, or perhaps a panel of teachers can select the best products and ads.

HOW DID IT GET HERE?

Grades 4–8

"How did it get here?" allows students to work in reverse. In other words students work backwards from finished product to raw materials in order to trace the development of the product. This activity encourages students to think holistically about the development process.

Objectives
- To develop an appreciation for the work involved in the products that surround us.
- To diagram processes involved in developing a product that is commonly used.

Materials
- Poster board.
- Markers.
- Pencils and eraser.
- Ruler.
- Reference material: magazines, encyclopedias, nonfiction books, textbooks, and so on.

Procedure
- As part of a unit on material resources, this activity is valuable to show the complex train of processes used to make an everyday product.
- It may be done as a group or solo project. It could be a project assigned for outside of class, or class time may be given.
- Develop a list of products we use. The list may include: pencils, gasoline, safety pins, frozen corn, cereal, and so on. Have each student or team select one product to trace. A sample sequence may be done to ensure that students are aware of the need to ask questions.

Evaluation

- How well did the students think in reverse? Did the best students develop a sequence of development that was logical and accurate? Was an appreciation for products established?

YOUR COAT OF ARMS

Grades 4–6

This activity involves using symbols to express personal meaning. Many times, thoughts can be expressed more effectively in visual rather than written form. This activity stimulates students to think visually on a personal subject.

Objective
- To use symbols in a coat of arms to express one's positive qualities.

Materials
- Ditto of shield and questions to be used.
- Markers, crayons, pencil, eraser.

Procedure
- Explain to students what a coat of arms is, how it was used, and that living up to one's family history puts pressure on many adults and children. This provides an opportunity for the students to consider what they expect of themselves and what good they see in themselves.
- They are to create their family shields according to the following:
  1. Three of their best qualities.
  2. Have them draw a symbol to represent something they do well.
  3. Have them draw a symbol to represent an important event in their lives.
  4. Have them make up a symbol to represent an important event in their family histories.
  5. Have them draw something that represents what they hope to accomplish in their lifetimes.

Alternative

· Or, if preferred, students may design their own coats of arms.
· The shield may be used as a format for reporting a biography of a relative, most-admired person, and so on.

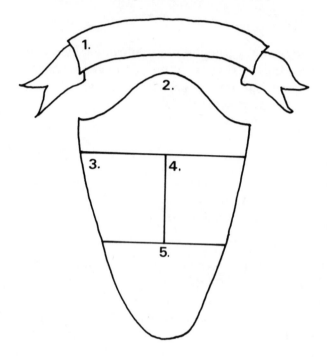

MORE THAN A DAY OFF

Grades 3–8

After three or four years of school, students know the basics about people and events celebrated during the school year. The following multimedia activity encourages students to look for more information, the kind of knowledge that adds a greater dimension to our understanding of holidays.

Objectives
- To find significant, but little-known facts that add to the comprehension of a holiday or a person who is honored on a special day.

Materials
- Library resources.
- Audiovisual materials.
- Other materials, to be determined by students.

Procedure
- This activity can be done in groups of four or five students, with each group taking a particular holiday or person. The task may be done by all groups at the same time and then used on the appropriate occasion. Or, a group can be pulled together and started about two weeks before the holiday.
- The groups are required to find at least four facts that are not commonly presented in reference to their particular holiday. Students must be able to provide some explanation of their findings, either in paragraphs, a rhyme, song, film, picture shows, booklets, and so on. Method of presentation may be determined by the group.
- A class discussion and list of what constitutes "basic facts" about the holiday is helpful. Also, there might be some form of checking

on the students after the presentation to see what they understood from their presentation.

Evaluation

· The students can be evaluated on all facets of their presentation.

CELEBRATION

Grades 4–9

It seems that around February, time goes very slowly in school. There are many ways to perk things up. Teachers have invented most of them. It seems only fair to give students a chance to try it. This exercise provides students with an opportunity to develop a little mythology of their own and to create a holiday to be celebrated sometime in midwinter.

Objectives
- To name and describe a new midwinter holiday celebration.
- To develop a history for this holiday celebration.

Materials
- A library for resource material.

Procedure
- By Christmas time, students have already heard the lore of four or more holidays. They will have some exposure to folk tales, mythology, and history. With this background and available reference materials, students are to be given time to create their own holiday.
- The teacher may request that specific kinds of information be developed, such as:
  Name of holiday _____
  Reason for celebration _____
  Date of celebration _____
  Is this related to any other historical event? If so, what? ___
- What is the story behind this holiday? (Include who was involved, what happened, what was important.) We want details, details. . . .
  Why should we consider this to be an important day?
  What activities should be used for this celebration?

- The final result of this could be a student vote on one holiday they would like to celebrate.
- For elementary students, there may be a need to work through this development together once in an abbreviated form to help them get started.
- A list of reasons for celebrating holidays would be helpful for students at any level.

CHAPTER SEVEN

Content Area Activities
9–12

The age, abilities, and interests of junior-high and high-school students open new paths of discovery. The use of various media is possible and wonderful for younger students; it is infinitely more so in the hands of students who have developed the skills and technical abilities to use media to maximum benefit. Of course, even very young students, given the optimal environment that encourages them to manipulate and experiment with a variety of media will develop these skills early, but adolescents have the added maturity to refine their interests.

During their early years, children seem primed for exploring and celebrating the various modes of learning. This is not to say that the very young do not have preferences; indeed, the whole theory of this book is that our innate biology helps structure our unique methods of processing reality. But due to brain development (see chapter 3), young children readily leap from interest to interest and method to method if given the opportunity.

By adolescence, a student has usually refined his or her interests. Whether his or her selection is truly a reflection of personal inclinations and inner needs, or an imposed decision (directly or indirectly due to the structure of the student's previous education) may have a great deal to do with how the student has learned to think. For example, do more males tend to enter the medical field because of social conditioning or because of the way in which the sciences are taught? Because visual–spatial development seems to be stronger in males, do they respond to laboratory learning, common to the sciences, more avidly than females? If different methods were used to teach the sciences, would there be a higher proportion of female doctors?

The answer is speculative, but logical. It would seem to make sense to present knowledge in every way possible in order to meet the needs of every student. But, by the time a student is in high school, he or she may be so dependent upon one mode of learning that it is very difficult for that student even to try different approaches or even subjects which favor the type of thinking to which the student is unaccustomed.

At this point, it takes the creative efforts of teachers working together to help relax the rigidity of the older student. In a traditional American high school, this is not an easy task. The system itself is a product of logical thinking, organized into departments so that students can be taught by specialists in the different subjects offered. While this is admirable and often very effective, it is also not as effective as it could be. A typical high school has very few students who fully use the specialized skills of their teachers. A more common situation is a classroom full of students "doing time," plugging through the courses they dislike for the sake of the few courses they excel in or enjoy. Or, even worse, one will see students who are totally uninterested in school, therefore causing discipline problems.

While it is too simplistic to say that boredom and failure in school is a direct result of the over-logical approach we have toward schooling, there is evidence to indicate that a more holistic approach might be a viable answer.

A graphic illustration can be seen by the example of what happens when novels are made into films. Film is a medium that relies heavily on the visual–spatial skills of the right hemisphere. Logic and language are involved, but the experience of a film can be justly said to be more holistic than the experience of a novel. Yet when a film based on a novel is successful, the sales of the book on which it is based increase dramatically. A great deal of this has to do with the marketing; the photograph, say, of Robert Redford as Jay Gatsby on the cover of a paperback reissue undoubtedly helps sales of *The Great Gatsby*. But something had to spark the nonreader to enter the bookstore before he could see the appealing dustcover.

An even more interesting phenomenon is a film company that produces a film first, and then, because of public demand, commissions a writer to turn the script into a novel. In both cases, contact with a more holistic approach encouraged contact with a more logical experience. The same phenomenon could occur in our schools.

It is far easier to sit at the keyboard of a typewriter and recommend a course of action than it is for a system entrenched in its own structure to change. Teachers often have very few choices concerning curriculum or even methodology. The philosophy of the school, the type of students, the attitudes of the parents and fellow teachers can all affect how any one teacher will direct his or her own classroom. If you teach in a situation that is not supportive of any deviation from a prescribed norm, for example, a school with a strong back-to-basics philosophy, there are still techniques and tools you can use on a personal basis. On the other hand, there are schools where some experimentation is feasible and welcome. Your situation will probably fall somewhere between the two. The ideas that follow will attempt to meet both needs. The suggestions presented are general because the specialized nature of high-school subjects requires adaptation by the person doing the actual teaching.

General Ideas for Any Situation, No Matter How Limiting A Situation

If you are tied to five books you must teach in your sophomore English class, or if your supervisor requires daily quizzes in your geometry class, there are still ways to balance the imposed linear structure. The area you have the most control over is your manner of presentation. The overwhelming reliance upon verbal instruction is a good place to initiate change. Before even thinking of new strategies, it might be beneficial, and probably surprising, to verify exactly how much time you spend talking. Record some class session unobtrusively and determine the percentage of class time you spend talking. The same diagnosis should be applied to your written instructions to students. How many worksheets do you distribute each week? How many pages of reading material?

The next step is to determine how much change you want to initiate. You could take a very logical approach and determine that you want to spend 25 percent less time talking, or, probably more realistic, you could use a more intuitive method, and get the feel of using alternative methods of instruction. Even the conscious realization that you want to reduce verbal instruction will help achieve more of a balance.

The next step is more difficult, for both you and your students. Alternatives to time-worn traditional teaching methods are hard to develop and often time-consuming, at least initially. Reading and speaking have probably evolved as the standard teaching methods because they are, or at least seem to be, time efficient. The problem is that they often do not work for every student. Such methods also value efficiency over other desired ends such as understanding or problem solving. As a teacher, you must develop new strategies for presenting and exploring your subject matter.

Students who have spent seven or eight years in a traditional system will find changes disconcerting, even those that promise to relieve boredom. As students are encouraged to deal with alternative ways of thinking and processing information, their behavior may reflect the changes. Discipline may be haywire for a while. It is a natural reaction to the loss of security and should be expected and taken into account when planning.

Exactly what are some of the alternative strategies available? A great deal depends on your subject matter. Initially, a good rule of thumb is to introduce as many visuals as possible. This may seem obvious, but it is rarely used to the extent where it becomes a real teaching tool. Obviously a geometry teacher draws diagrams, but these are usually accompanied with verbal proof. What if students were greeted one day with a lyric film on architecture, emphasizing the geometric shapes in classical buildings? With no verbal introduction and no follow-up explanation, the class would certainly be puzzled. But almost just as certainly, questions would follow, and these, if handled correctly, could lead into other explorations of the same nature. Learning theorems would still be very much a part of the class, but such variations or presentations could lead to a more complete understanding of what geometry actually is.

Providing experiences for the students to participate in rather than read about is another route open to the classroom teacher. Thus, an English teacher could call a Monday "Elizabethan Day" nd require the class to dress and speak in the authentic style of the period. A biology class could expereince the thrill an archaeologist eels when discovering an ancient skeleton, even if it means the eacher has to spend an evening planting a chicken skeleton in the ootball field. Rather than reading about the scientific process of excavating, re-creating and dating bones, the students could do it hemselves.

Again, such projects encourage development of both linear and olistic processes. Research will almost always lead the student to ooks and nondirected situations which will require brainstorming nd nonlogical approaches.

In spite of the overwhelming reliance on linear subjects in our chools, some subjects are by nature very visually oriented and could se a dose of logic to round out the student's experience. Verbal liscussions and lectures on the history of the development of painting could put some needed structure into a freshman fine arts class hat has turned into a dabbling session. The same applies to a vocal music class. A mathematical analysis of the Bach chorale that the lass has been practicing for weeks might give students the added mpetus to master its complexity.

Many other media besides the pencil and paper are available to eachers and students. Video equipment, tape recorders, cameras, musical instruments, modelling clay, and bread dough are all materiuls that can be used to help investigate a subject.

Evaluations need not be written or verbal. The required weekly vocabulary test would still require the student to learn definitions if ie or she had to create a collage illustrating the meaning of one issigned word during the class session the day of the test.

Devising alternative teaching strategies need not be a lonely or overwhelming task. Most of us are products of a lopsided education ourselves, and may find it difficult to create new ways to present naterial. In most high schools, the resources are as near as the aculty lounge. If you know nothing about visual arts but are interested in using more visual methods in your classroom, ask the art eacher for suggestions, or maybe even painting lessons. The drama eacher will certainly be able to help with methods of presentation, especially in the areas of body language and oral communication. A shop teacher may want to consult the composition teacher to find a better way of teaching organization or sequencing to help students in his visually oriented class become more analytic in their approach.

After trying a few new techniques, use your own intuitive feelings and some verifiable evaluation techniques to determine whether your new methods are working. If you are uncomfortable with the changes after giving them a sufficient chance, retrench and think some more. There are no right or wrong ways to teach or learn. There is only the process. Just keep in mind that a good balancing act needs a lot of practice.

Some Ideas for Curriculum Development

While individual teachers can begin to encourage more balanced thought in their own classrooms, they are probably limited by curriculum directives in their desire to offer their students a variety of experiences. If the student spends but one of the five or six class periods in a typical high-school day with a teacher who believes that more nonverbal, holistic experiences are necessary, the impact upon the student will be minor. Such a situation may even make the concerned teacher's job more difficult because of the insecurity students may initially feel in response to the new techniques. If the teacher finds himself among skeptical or even somewhat hostile colleagues who support the students' initial balkiness, he might as well be swimming up river with a rock tied around his waist.

This is not to say that individual teachers have no power to encourage more balanced thinking by techniques and methods within their own classrooms, but their effectiveness will be limited at best. A much more effective approach would be to adapt the curriculum to meet the special needs of both types of thinking rather than providing students with a lopsided helping of overly rational course offerings.

At this point, it is not redundant to emphasize that a more balanced education usually provides a synergistic effect in development, rather than watering down the effects of a more specialized education. Examples such as those in chapter nine illustrate that rational as well as holistic skills improve when the nonverbal side of the brain is addressed in addition to the logical side. Because, at least on a superficial level, it appears that our society demands competence in the logical–rational skills over the more ambiguous holistic skills, we hesitate to interfere with anything that will impede learning in those areas. Currently, such subjects as art and music are "gravy," nice but not necessary, while the "meat and potatoes" courses like reading and math are seen as necessary for survival. The logical approach is to concentrate on that which seems important and to ignore the rest. As is often the case, the purely one-sided answer is often less effective than the answer arrived at by a more balanced approach. The back-to-basics movement is a classic example of this. Excluding the nonrational courses in order to concentrate upon the logical, survival skills has not effectively produced students who are more competent in the rational skills.

Enough said on the topic. If you as a reader did not believe that balance in the classroom is important, you probably would have put this book down long ago.

A Balanced Curriculum

The reality of changing a curriculum in a typical school which has to answer to state, federal, and (more binding, perhaps) traditional guidelines, is as probable as passing a school tax levy. Small successes, however, can encourage larger gains. If any real educational changes are to be evidenced from brain research, they will come slowly. Thus the following plan is an example of how a traditional junior high or high school might initiate a more balanced curriculum.

The first step would be to provide some in-service awareness courses for the faculty. A solid understanding of the necessity for a balanced curriculum, and some opportunity to see how one's own subject can be presented in a more balanced way should precede any major undertakings. This need not be expensive or even require outside consultants. If a core group of interested teachers and/or administrators prepare themselves, they could in turn supervise this awareness process. An ideal situation would be to make a commitment to balancing the curriculum and teaching methods at the beginning of the school year. Then faculty meetings, departmental meetings, in-service days, and budgets could all be used to further the goal. With an entire staff aware and concerned, new ideas should be commonplace.

The students' role in this should not be passive. The theories behind the new changes they will experience should prove fascinating and motivating. Such all-school projects tend to create an enthusiasm known (at least on the basketball court and football field) as school spirit. The benefit of this type of motivator is that it is integral to the program and it has something for everybody. All students will be involved in situations with which they are familiar and unfamiliar. No one area should be valued over another; therefore, the successes experienced in all subjects will be true successes. Because the curriculum will be more balanced, students who excel in the areas that are traditionally neglected or not respected should gain in self-respect.

Students should also grow in self-awareness through the emphasis placed on learning styles. They will be encouraged to discover their preferred modes of learning and to use the materials and media that will best meet their needs. The approach to this discovery process should be both formal and intuitive. A schoolwide evaluation could be made using one of the inventories mentioned in chapter five. But the student's own interests and intuitive opinions should be considered just as valid.

Actual change in the curriculum is something that will happen more slowly. Solid evidence of success will probably be needed before district guidelines would allow course requirements and budgets to reflect the needs of a balanced curriculum. The following is an idea for a "test case" or opportunity for a school to "dip its toe in the water" before plunging into change.

In many districts, there is a week or two of days set aside for testing or special activities. Instead of spreading these days out, they could be grouped to form a minisemester of one or two weeks duration. In these two weeks, students would be offered a curriculum that would include as the basics reading and art, and science and music. To provide a more effective experience, a general theme will unify the two weeks, giving the students a goal and solidifying the experience. This will also allow for a variety of evaluation techniques to be employed.

For example, a current issue such as nuclear energy or endangered species could become the preoccupation of the school for two weeks. Or the theme could be a film, a topic such as osmosis, or a work of art. For clarity, let's say that the play *Romeo and Juliet* will be the unifying experience for the plan outlined here. Because this is a play that is often taught in high school, it will also serve as a comparison to illustrate what is different and, in many cases, the same in a traditional curriculum and a more balanced approach.

From the beginning it should be clear that the purpose is not to produce a stage version of the play. That may be one approach chosen, but it is not the single desired outcome. Rather, the process is what is important, not the product. If anything, the goal is to understand the play through whatever media and methods will best allow for it.

Each subject area will deal with *Romeo and Juliet* in some way. This may seem tricky when it comes to biology or chemistry, yet there are various approaches that could be taken. If the science teacher wanted to emphasize, for example, the scientific method, and illustrate how a scientist thinks through a hypothesis, he might do an analytic study of the play. How would the end have been different if Romeo had encountered each situation through a hypothesis-proof situation? Another approach might be to study the botony mentioned in the play, or to do a chemical analysis of the herbs the friar used.

The English teacher need not rest on his laurels just because the play falls into his territory. If anything, he should make a rule not to teach the play as he has on previous occasions. If his technique was for the classes to read the play and then view the film, he might reverse the order. Or perhaps the classes could read the first two acts, then view the film version of the rest of the play. He might use mime or music to meet his objectives. In any case, he should try to reach clearly both sides of the brain in his methods and content.

It is interesting to note that such an arrangement needs cross-disciplinary cooperation. In fact, this is the only way for a balanced curriculum to work. To merely equal time allotments of the more holistic courses is to deny that a person needs to learn to think alternatively in every facet of his life. One does not turn off rational skills when entering the art studio any more than one's intuitive insight in the mathematics laboratory. While labeling courses art–literature could become a bureaucratic nightmare, the open flow between and among traditional disciplines must be encouraged.

The following are some more ideas which teachers in various disciplines use for the school project:

Art: Create masks, costumes, visual personality sketches.

Music: Analytic study of Elizabethan music; compose a piece in the Elizabethan style.

Theatre: Replicate a Shakespearean production, using the methods an Elizabethan actor would have used.

Language: Be a Frenchman or a Spaniard of the period, investigate literature with similar themes in the language of study.

History/Social Science: Analyze the social conditions that created the crisis in *Romeo and Juliet.* Be an authentic Elizabethan for a day.

Physics: Create a set for a production using intricate forces, pulleys, and levers.

The experiences planned for the classroom should be a combined planning effort by all of those involved. Cross-disciplinary involvement is encouraged, either on a consultant basis or in the experience. Some new unplanned-for things might happen and should be allowed; they are part of the process. Students should have some choice of course offerings, with the stipulation that they must take at least two courses from a rationally oriented discipline and two courses from a more holistically oriented one, out of a total of five.

Evaluation of the minisemester should occur in a balanced way also. Traditional, rational pretest–post-test studies might be done, testing everything from understanding of the material covered to attitude changes. Product-oriented evaluation can be done, such as displays of art work, films, or publications produced by the students.

Discussions of general feelings about the experience should be considered valid data.

The outcome may lead to more such experiences or to more permanent changes. Or it may prove so overwhelming as to discourage change. To meet the needs of both sides of the brain is not a neat and orderly experience. There are no right answers, only human answers.

CHAPTER EIGHT

The Next Step: Curriculum Development

Thus far we have summarized some recent findings in the area of brain research and have suggested classroom activities based on the hemispheric model. Often the question is asked: "How can we link these classroom activities into a program or curriculum?" The answer to this question depends upon curriculum development and the role of the instructional leader.

Curriculum Development

Several references have been made to the two modes of thinking associated with the hemispheres of the brain. This concept is the key to the kind of curriculum development that is responsive to the current findings in brain research. As educators develop curricula, they should keep in mind the hemispheric concept in addition to other findings from brain research. Then it will be possible to plan a balanced course of study and instructional strategies. The following method is suggested as a step-by-step process for implementing the kind of curriculum that is based on brain-related strategies.

I. Exploration of Research

The first step is to acquire the knowledge base and rationale for brain-related curriculum development. This book provides a beginning; for additional information see the bibliography. You will want to explore other models that seek to explain the functioning of the brain, especially those that are of particular interest in your teaching–learning situation. Developing this knowledge base about brain functioning is extremely important.

II. Needs Assessment

The second step in curriculum development is to gain some understanding of the status of your current curriculum as it relates to hemispheric processes. The assessment also indicates what should be done and generates interest among the teachers in the school. This step can be carried out through a needs-assessment survey or through interviews conducted by the instructional leader. At the conclusion of this step, the developer has a data base for initiating relevant goals and objectives.

III. Goals and Objectives

After determining needs and interests, step three is to establish goals and objectives. These may relate to balancing the curriculum, further exploration of brain research, or developing classroom applications. The goals and objectives should be established collaboratively and should be accepted and supported by those who participate. They should provide focus and direction to the development of the curriculum and be related to those concerns that have come about through an understanding of current findings in brain research.

IV. Delivery System

In the fourth step, the instructional leader determines how to carry out the objectives and reach the goals. Will consultant services and/or materials on brain studies be provided for the teachers? Who will do the writing of the curriculum, testing, and so on? In general, this step leads the participants to think through the process of achieving the goals in curriculum development and to establish a time-line.

V. Evaluation

As part of the planning process, an evaluation model should be selected and used to determine the effectiveness of the new plan involving those changes made to achieve a more balanced curriculum. The collected data can be used to disseminate the results of your efforts by sharing the data with others in the district or state or in education journals. Evaluation can also provide suggestions for making improvements during the formative stages of your project;

at the end, it will give you evidence as to whether or not you met your goals.

VI. *Institutional Adoption*

The last step in the program development process assures that the effective products of the effort are retained in the system. This is accomplished by making the necessary changes in the program and budget and by providing up-to-date information to key people who make decisions regarding the curriculum.

As presented in the preceding paragraphs, the program development process for making curricula responsive to brain research appears lock-stepped and compartmentalized. In practice, however, many of the steps overlap, occur simultaneously, or are shifted. So, the process should be viewed as a flexible blueprint from which to operate in order to achieve the goals and objectives of program development and to bring about permanent benefits from such development.

Role of Instructional Leader

The key player in developing programs is the instructional leader or curriculum specialist. This person can use the development plan to unify and enhance activities based on the hemispheric brain theory. In following this plan, the school or district will initiate the development of curricular programs that employ classroom applications based on research into the functioning of the brain. As a result, curricula and instructional strategies become congruent with the discoveries of how the brain functions in teaching and learning. This union will provide increased effectiveness for schools.

Holistic Schooling

It was stated previously that school curricula tend to suppress the holistic, simultaneous, and intuitive mode of consciousness. The basic subjects in school have long been considered the primarily linear subjects of reading, writing, and mathematics, to the neglect of nonlinear subjects such as art, dance, and media studies. The back-to-basics movement is a reemphasizing of the linear mode of thought. It assumes that concentration on reading, writing, and mathematics will develop competent individuals. In line with the hemispheric specialization theory, however, students will only be half-developed. In the curriculum, a fourth component is needed (in addition to reading, writing, and mathematics) to develop the simultaneous and metaphoric processes. Formal schooling must stress both linear and holistic modes of consciousness.

Individualized education and confluent education are two examples of approaches in which the holistic mode is utilized in balance with the linear mode. The individualized classroom is flexible, with space divided into learning centers rather than one fixed, homogeneous unit. Individually or in groups, students are permitted to explore the classroom environment and select their learning activities. Multimedia resources abound; there is no reliance on one particular medium. The teacher's instruction is usually on a one-to-one basis or with small groups rather than with the entire class. The individualized-instruction classroom allows students to develop their interests and to follow their intuition as the teacher assists in constructing an individualized curriculum for each one. In addition to learning the basics, students develop functions associated with the right hemisphere of the brain through activities that emphasize holistic and simultaneous approaches.

Confluent education emphasizes the integration of the affective and cognitive domains. The affective domain involves values, emotions, and attitudes. The cognitive domain includes the intellectual processes of an individual, what and how a person learns. Confluent education blends the intellectual and emotional factors in learning and teaching. This blending is often parallel to the integration of the activities associated with the right and left hemispheres.

Another curriculum area that attempts to integrate the two modes of consciousness is instructional media. Visual media stress the spatial and simultaneous processes of the right hemisphere and encourage thinking visually. In addition, the sequencing involved in most visual media (e.g., action in films, order of slides in slide–tape presentations) enhances the integration of the functions of the right and left hemisheres. Media, which are applicable to most teaching–learning situations, use the functions of both hemispheres.

Summary

This chapter discussed the question of what is next in terms of program or curriculum development based on current findings in brain research. In view of the findings, it seems appropriate to link some of the classroom applications of the hemispheric theory with curriculum designs and programs. Such programs can form the foundation for further linkages and applications of cerebral research findings as they become available. A step-by-step method was suggested to develop programs. Some sample programs were presented. This procedure will provide the basis for implementing future results from brain research, some of which we look at next.

CHAPTER NINE

Exploring the Frontiers of Learning

We have presented some of the current theories about brain functioning. They contain exciting information that some day may truly revolutionize the field of education and how we think about the practice of teaching and learning. We have also given some classroom applications that are suggested by the hemispheric specialization of the brain. In this chapter, we want to speculate about the future: Where will the increased knowledge about the brain lead educators? This will be supplemented (in chapter ten) by a list of resources that will help you gain additional knowledge about brain research and stimulate your thinking about the educational applications of such research.

As a prelude to your exploration of the implications of brain research for your classroom, let us consider some general concepts about the meaning of brain research for your particular situation.

The Evolution of Consciousness

We have discussed the dominance of the linear–sequential mode of consciousness both in and out of school. We expressed the opinion that the linear–sequential mode is an incomplete way of viewing reality. What is needed is a balanced and integrated approach that utilizes both modes of consciousness (the holistic, simultaneous, and intuitive in addition to the linear–sequential). When this occurs, the next step is integration between the two modes. The following model uses both modes of thinking, individually as needed and jointly when appropriate. This practice provides additional flexibility, increased awareness, and fuller brain utilization.

Integration of the Modes

As classroom practice succeeds in helping youngsters use the functions of both hemispheres of the brain, an integration of functions occurs, exhibiting traits of unity, synthesis, and balance. Inappropriate and fragmented approaches to learning and schooling are replaced by those which are holistic and integrated. The integrated mode provides a balanced approach that was previously lacking.

Grady & Luecke (Phi Delta Kappa Fastback #108, *Education and the Brain*) speculated that the use of both modes of consciousness or thinking in learning results in a synergetic mode of consciousness which is reserved for peak experiences rather than everyday experiences. This concept may be represented by the following diagram.

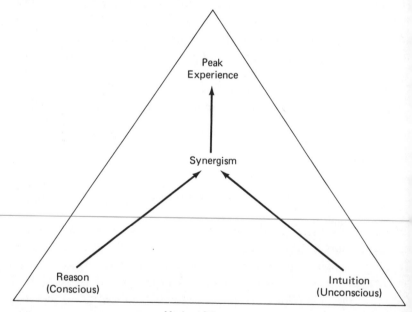

Modes of Awareness

The unconscious level (in the triangle) is indicated by the right-hemispheric function of intuition. The theory regarding this function is not new, but the intent is to stress the value of right-hemispheric functions and to practice and utilize them. As the usage of the right-hemispheric functions increases along with the already practiced and valued functions of the left hemisphere (indicated in the diagram by reason), there will be increased occurrences of the synergetic mode of consciousness. The ultimate event comes about when reason and intuition are synchronized in those rare, synergetic moments that produce peak experiences. A person may write effective rhymes and rhythms but lack the intuitive insights that make one poet great and another mediocre. It is the combination of the rational–linear skills and intuitive insights which produces great poetry through synergetic experiences.

While it is probably true that the synergetic mode of consciousness operates infrequently, its occurrence produces exhilarating results. The catalyst which makes it possible is the development of the previously neglected and undervalued right hemisphere. An increase in traditional formal schooling is not what is needed in this development. Instead, nonlinear processes must have a place in the curriculum or students must search for them outside of the formal school setting.

Other Developments

In the fast-moving area of brain research, other recent discoveries related to education include the following. Sandra Witelson, writing in *Science* (January 1977), suggests that children with developmental reading difficulties may have spatial functioning represented in both hemispheres, not only the right. She reported that such students have language lateralized in the left hemisphere, which is typical, but that left-hemisphere language processes are interfered with by spatial functioning in both hemispheres. This situation causes a deficiency in the children's ability to perform sequential, cognitive tasks such as phonetic interpretation. Instead, the students rely on spatial strategies which are not sufficient to perform the task. She says that children with reading difficulties learned to comprehend Chinese logographs which use visual, holistic processing rather than sequential functions. Perhaps children with reading difficulties need instruction that employs the functions of both hemispheres in order to learn to read.

Along the same line of thought, *Brain Mind Bulletin* (June 1, 1981) reported on a Los Angeles teacher who has taught trainable mentally retarded children to read thousands of words in sign language before they read them in print. Phil Brody used sign language to teach them the alphabet, a task they had not accomplished previously. He then started to teach them words, after which they started to read and became more verbal. His method relies mostly on sight recognition rather than phonics. Brody believes that signing may be an intermediate step, based on the students' basic strength and ability, that helps them use hemispheric processes that bridge the gap to verbal skills.

New evidence from hemispheric-specialization research suggests that the left hemisphere specializes in fine resolution operations and the right hemisphere specializes in gross resolution operations. Both hemispheres can analyze, but the left does a finer job. This finding sheds new light on the interpretation that the left hemisphere is analytical and the right is holistic. In her experiments, Justine Sergent of McGill University found that the primary difference in hemispheric specialization was in the frequency or fineness of detail of incoming information (*Brain Mind Bulletin*, March 28, 1983). The right hemisphere, she believes, is a quick study, a good guesser, faster or more accurate than the left when time is short or image quality is poor. The left gives a fine resolution when it has enough time and information. The right brain provides the framework for the left brain's more refined operations.

Jerry Levy of the University of Chicago is quoted in the May 9, 1983 edition of the *Brain Mind Bulletin* as saying that "normal brains are built to be challenged. They operate at optimal levels only when cognitive processing requirements are of sufficient complexity to activate both sides of the brain." According to Levy's analysis, in the 1960s the humanistic approach favored by many educators emphasized a "non-threatening setting for learning. But a non-threatening environment should not mean a non-challenging one. Challenges are what appear to engage the whole brain, generate excitement and provide the substrate for optimal learning. . . .

Educationally this means that simple, repetitive, and uninteresting problems would be poorly learned with little benefit for either side of the brain."

Levy added that the corpus callosum plays a role in facilitating arousal of both hemispheres. Tasks requiring interhemispheric communication appear to engage strongly both hemispheres. "If this in turn promotes optimal functioning, people should be able to perform dual tasks as well as or better than single tasks." Thus, it seems that implementing the curriculum projects suggested in this book will provide a beginning for using brain research results in ways that will enchance learning and stimulate the brain.

A last note concerns the business community. In addition to educators using results from brain research, people such as Dudley Lynch of Brain Technologies Corporation in Lawton, Oklahoma, and Ned Hermann, a New York management educator, are applying research efforts to business. Lynch talks about mind styles for management in order to improve the chances that companies have an employee–job match that is appropriate and lasting. If this match is appropriate, the business mind can work its way toward a style suited to understanding and responding to contemporary problems.

Ned Hermann uses a test to determine hemispheric dominance. He then gathers a mix of people to function as a whole brain. They work jointly and individually to develop solutions to problems of personal interest. In this way, Hermann provides for the integration of left- and right-hemispheric processes in order to reach novel solutions to problems.

These developments and others will provide a challenging and productive environment for educators. We believe that brain research will provide the most helpful knowledge for educators during the remainder of this century as we attempt to improve schooling.

A Basis for a Theory of Education

In addition to the rewards to be gained from an increased understanding of hemispheric specialization and other functions of the brain, a larger benefit will be the development of a theory or foundational basis for teaching and learning. Although there is evidence to support the theory that learning takes place in the brain, we do not have a complete understanding of how the brain functions and consequently have not been able to develop a sound foundation for a theory of learning. If brain research continues to reveal the mysteries of the brain and its functions in relation to learning, teaching, and memory, we will know more about how learning occurs and can then build an educational system based on physiological data. This system could be, for the first time, educationally sound in relation to our knowledge about how the brain functions. The benefit for children will be enormous, since education will enter a new era as the brain becomes a basis for a theory of learning.

Conclusion

We are embarking on an exciting phase in education marked by recent advances in the neurosciences. Soon we will have the knowledge to form a scientific basis for the practice of teaching and learning. This new knowledge will enable educators to make quantum leaps in improving classroom instruction. We urge you to explore relevant studies coming from the neurosciences and consider their significance in terms of applications for the classroom. Brain research requires a multidisciplinary approach. Educators must take part in the studies if researchers are to comprehend fully the functions of the brain. We hope that this book provides an impetus for you to study research on the brain and apply the findings to your classroom.

Bibliography

The following references were selected to aid educators who wish to pursue additional information about the brain, seek more in-depth knowledge about particular aspects of cerebral research, or further their knowledge about classroom applications.

The references have been placed in categories to assist the reader in selecting appropriate resources.

Hemispheric Specialization of the Brain
Early Research

Bogen, Joseph E. 1969. The other side of the brain. *Bulletin of the Los Angeles Neurological Society* 34, 1:73–105, 11:135–62; 111: 191–220.

Bogen, Joseph E., E. D. Fisher, and P. J. Vogel. 1965. Cerebral commissurotomy. *Journal of the American Medical Association* 194:1328–1329.

Gazzaniga, Michael S., Joseph E. Bogen, and Roger W. Sperry. 1965. Observations on visual perception after disconnexion of the cerebral hemispheres in man. *Brain* 88, (Part 2):221–236.

Gazzaniga, Michael S., Joseph E. Bogen, and Roger W. Sperry. 1962. Some functional effects of sectioning the cerebral commissures in man. *Proceedings of the National Academy of Sciences* 48: 1765–1769.

Gazzaniga, Michael S., and Roger W. Sperry. 1967. Language after section of the cerebral commissures. *Brain* 90, (Part 1):131–148.

Mountcastle, Vernon B., (ed.). *Conference on hemispheric relations and cerebral dominance.* Baltimore: The Johns Hopkins Press, 1962.

Sperry, Roger W. 1964. The great cerebral commissure. *Scientific American* 210 (January):42–52.

Sperry, Roger W. 1961. Cerebral organization and behavior. *Science* 133:- 1749–1757.

General Readings
Books

Arnheim, Rudolf. *Visual thinking.* Los Angeles: University of California Press, 1969.

———. *The brain, a Scientific American book.* San Francisco: W. H. Freeman and Company, 1979.

Brown, Barbara B. *Supermind: The ultimate energy.* New York: Harper & Row, 1980.

Bruner, Jerome. *On knowing, essays for the left hand.* Cambridge: Harvard University Press, 1966.

Chall, Jeanne, and Allan Mirsky (eds.). *Education and the brain.* The seventy-seventh yearbook of the National Society for the Study of Education. Chicago: University of Chicago Press, 1978.

Corballis, M. C., and I. L. Beale. *The psychology of left and right.* Hillsdale, N.J.: Erlbaum, 1976.

Dimond, S. J., and D. A. Blizard (eds.). *Evolution and lateralization of the brain.* New York: New York Academy of Sciences, 1977.

Edwards, Betty. *Drawing on the right side of the brain.* Los Angeles: J. P. Tarcher, Inc., 1979.

Ferguson, Marilyn. *The brain revolution.* New York: Taplinger, 1973.

Fincher, J. *Sinister people.* New York: Putnam's, 1977.

Gardener, Howard. *The shattered mind: The person after brain damage.* New York: Alfred A. Knopf, 1975.

Gazzaniga, Michael S. *The bisected brain.* New York: Appleton-Century-Crofts, 1970.

Gazzaniga, Michael S., and Joseph E. Leder. *The integrated mind.* New York: Plenum Press, 1978.

Geschwind, Norman. *Selected papers on language and the brain.* Boston: D. Reidel Publishing, 1974.

Grady, Michael P., and Emily A. Luecke. *Education and the brain.* Bloomington, Ind.: Phi Delta Kappa Foundation (#108), 1978.

Hart, Leslie. *How the brain works.* New York: Basic Books, 1975.

Hart, Leslie A. *Human brain and human learning.* New York: Longman, 1983.

Jaynes, Julian. *The origin of consciousness in the breakdown of the bicameral mind.* Boston: Houghton Mifflin, 1976.

Lee, Philip R., et al. *Symposium on consciousness.* New York: Viking Press, 1976.

McKim, Robert H. *Experiences in visual thinking.* Monterey, California: Brooks/Cole, 1972.

Ornstein, Robert E. *The mind field.* New York: Viking Press, 1976.

Ornstein, Robert E. *The psychology of consciousness.* San Francisco: W. H. Freeman, 1972.

Orton, S. T. *Reading, writing, and speech problems in children.* New York: Norton, 1937.

Popper, Karl R., and John C. Eccles. *The self and its brain.* New York: Springer International, 1977.

Restak, Richard M. *The brain: The last frontier.* New York: Warner Books, 1979.

Rockefeller, David. *Coming to our senses: The significance of the arts for American education.* New York: McGraw-Hill, 1977.

Russell, Peter. *The brain book.* New York: E. P. Dutton, 1979.

Sagan, Carl. *The dragons of Eden.* New York: Ballantine, 1977.

Samples Bob. *The metaphoric mind.* Reading, Mass.: Addison-Wesley, 1976.

Samples, Robert, et al. *The whole school book: teaching and learning late in the twentieth century.* Reading, Mass.: Addison-Wesley, 1977.

Taylor, Gordon R. *The natural history of the mind.* New York: E. P. Dutton, 1979.

Wile, I. S. *Handedness: Right and left.* Boston: Lothrop, Lee & Shepard, 1934.

Wittrock, M. C., et al. *The human brain.* Englewood Cliffs, New Jersey: Prentice-Hall, Inc., 1977.

Wittrock, M. C. *The brain and psychology.* New York: Academic Press, 1980.

Articles

Bogen, Joseph E. 1975. Some educational aspects of hemispheric specialization. *UCLA Educator* 17:24–32. (This issue is on the hemispheric processes of the brain.)

Brain Mind Bulletin. Los Angeles: Interface Press. (Every three weeks)

Buchsbaum, Monte S. 1979. Tuning in on hemispheric dialogue. *Psychology Today* 12 (January): 100.

Corballis, Michael L. 1980. Laterality and myth. *American Psychologist* 35: 284–295.

——— 1981. Educational implications of recent brain research. (Symposium) *Educational Leadership* 39 (October): 6–13 ff.

Edwards, C. H. 1982. Brain function: Implications for schooling. *Contemporary Education* 53 (Winter): 58–60.

Ehrlichman, H., and A. Weinberger. 1978. Lateral eye movements and hemispheric asymmetry: A critical review. *Psychological Bulletin* 85: 1080–1101.

Frostig, M., and P. Maslow. 1979. Neuropsychological contributions to education. *Journal of Learning Disabilities* 12 (October): 538–51.

Galaburda, Albert M., Marrie LeMay, Thomas L. Kemper, and Norman Geschwind. 1978. Right–left asymmetries in the brain. *Science* 199: 852–856.

Gardner, Howard. 1981. How the split brain gets a joke. *Psychology Today* 15 (Feb.): 74–76 ff.

Gazzaniga, Michael S. 1967. The split brain in man. *Scientific American* 217 (August): 24–29.

Geschwind, Norman. 1979. Specialization of the human brain; learning capabilities and two cerebral hemispheres. *Scientific American* 241 (September): 180–2 ff. (This entire issue is about the brain.)

Goleman, Daniel. 1977. Split-brain psychology: Fad of the year. *Psychology Today* 11 (October): 89–90 ff.

Hardyck, C., and R. Haapanen. 1979. Educating both halves of the brain: Educational breakthrough or neuromythology? *Journal of School Psychology* 17 (Fall): 219–230.

Restak, R. M. 1981. His brain, her brain. (Interview; ed. by S. B. Zakariya), *Principal* 60 (May): 46–51.

Pribram, Karl, interviewed by Daniel Goleman. 1979. Holographic memory. *Psychology Today* 13 (February): 71–84.

Sperry, Roger W. 1968. Hemispheric disconnection and unity in conscious awareness. *American Psychologist* 23: 723–733.

———. 1969. A modified concept of consciousness. *Psychological Review* 76: 532–536.

Staley, F. A. 1980. Hemispheric brain research: A breakthrough for outdoor education. *Journal of Physical Education and Recreation* 51: 28–30.

Sylwester, Robert 1982. A child's brain. *Instructor* 92 (September): 91–96; 92 (October): 64–67; 92 (November-December): 44–46.

Tomlinson-Keasey, Carol, Ronald R. Kelly and John K. Burton. 1978. Hemispheric changes in information processing during development. *Developmental Psychology* 14: 214–223.

Wada, J. A., R. Clarke, and A. Hamm. 1975. Cerebral hemispheric asymmetry in humans. *Archives of Neurology* 32: 239–246.

Webster, William G., A. Dianne Thurber. 1978. Problem-solving strategies and manifest brain asymmetry. *Cortex* 14: 474–484.

Wenger, W. 1981. Creative creativity: Some strategies for developing specific areas of the brain and for working both sides together. *Journal of Creative Behavior* 15: 77–89.

Language

Buzan, Tony. *Use both sides of your brain.* New York: E. P. Dutton, 1976.

Cohen, G., and R. Freeman. Individual differences in reading strategies in relation to handedness and cerebral asymmetry. In J. Requin (ed.), *Attention and Performance VII.* Hillsdale, N.J.: Erlbaum, 1978.

Cunningham, M. D., and P. J. Murphy. 1981. Effects of bilateral EEG biofeedback on verbal, visual–spatial, and creative skills in learning disabled male adolescents. *Journal of Learning Disabilities* 14 (April): 204–8.

Dean, Raymond S. 1978. Cerebral laterality and reading comprehension. *Neuropsychologica* 16: 633–636.

Gazzaniga, Michael S. 1983. Right hemisphere language following brain bisection. *American Psychologist* 38: 525–537.

Gordon, Harold W. 1980. Cerebral organization in bilinguals: 1. Lateralization. *Brain & Language* 9: 255–268.

Harris, Albert J. 1979. Lateral dominance and reading disability. *Journal of Learning Disabilities* 12: 337–343.

Leong, G. K. Laterality and reading proficiency in children. *Reading Research Quarterly* 80, 15(2): 185–202.

Levy, Jere. 1983. Language, cognition, and the right hemisphere. *American Psychologist* 38: 538–541.

Naylor, Hilary. 1980. Reading disability and lateral asymmetry: An information-processing analysis. *Psychological Bulletin* 87: 531–545.

O'Leary, D. S. 1980. Developmental study of interhemispheric transfer in children aged five to ten. *Child Development* 51 (September): 743–750.

Tadanobu, T. 1979. Left cerebral hemisphere of the brain and the Japanese language. *Gifted Child Quarterly* 3 (Winter): 861–866.

Tallal, Paula. 1980. Auditory temporal perception, phonics, and reading disabilities in children. *Brain & Language* 9: 182–198.

Tomlinson-Keasey, Carol, and Ronald R. Kelly. 1978. The deaf child's symbolic world. *American Annals of the Deaf* 123: 452–459.

Vellutino, Frank R., William L. Bentley, and Forman Phillips. 1978. Interversus intra-hemispheric learning in dyslexic and normal readers. *Developmental Medicine and Child Neurology* 20: 71–80.

Witelson, S. F. 1977. Developmental dyslexia: Two right hemispheres and none left. *Science* 195: 309–311.

Handedness

Coren, S. and C. Porac. 1977. Fifty centuries of right-handedness: The historical record. *Science* 198: 631–632.

Hardyck, C., and L. F. Petrinovich. 1977. Left-handedness. *Psychological Bulletin* 84: 385–404.

Hacaen, H., and J. Sauget. 1971. Cerebral dominance in left-handed subjects. *Cortex* 7: 1948.

Peterson, J. M., and L. M. Lansky. 1974. Left-handedness among architects: Some facts and speculation. *Perceptual and Motor Skills* 38: 547–560.

Springer, Sally P., and Alan Searleman. 1978. Laterality in twins: The relationship between handedness and hemispheric asymmetry for speech. *Behavior Genetics* 8: 349–357.

Warren, J. M. 1980. Handedness and laterality in humans and other animals. *Physiological Psychology* 8: 351–359.

Wilson, D. 1972. Righthandedness. *The Canadian Journal* 75: 193–230.

Resources for Classroom Activities

Allison, Linda. *Blood and guts: A working guide to your own little insides.* New York: Little Brown, 1976.

Caney, Steve. *Steve Caney's kid's America.* New York: Workman Publishing, 1978.

Caney, Steve. *Steve Caney's toybook.* New York: Workman Publishing, 1972.

Canfield, Jack, and Harold C. Wells. *100 ways to enhance self-concept in the classroom.* Englewood Cliffs: Prentice Hall, 1976.

Carin, Arthur A., and Robert B. Sund. *Creative questioning and sensitive listening.* Charles E. Merrill Publishing Co., 1978.

Good Apple Publications, Carthage, Ill.: Good Apple Inc.

Kid's Stuff Publications, Nashville, Tenn.: Incentive Publications.

Lacock, Mary, and Gary Watson. *The fabric of mathematics.* Hayward, Calif.: Activity Resources, 1975.

Macaulay, David. *Cathedral: The story of its construction.* London: William Collins Sons and Co. Ltd., 1974.

National Wildlife Week Education Kits—Distributed to schools by the
    State department of Conservation or by contacting: National Wildlife
    Federation, 1412 16th St. NW Washington, D.C. 20036.

Raudsepp, Eugene and George P. Hough, Sr. *Creative growth games.* New
    York: Perigee Books, 1977.

Raudsepp, Eugene. *More creative games.* New York: Perigee Books, 1980.

Seymour, Dale et al. *Aftermath.* Palto Alto, Calif.: Creative Publications,
    1971.

Strongin, Herb. *Science on a shoestring.* Reading, Mass: Addison-Wesley
    Publishing Co., 1976.

Whittaker, Dora. *Move in on math: A four book graded course.* New York:
    Cuisenaire Co. of America, 1974.

Index

70.15
733t

DATE DUE

FEB 0 4	OC 20 '91	APR 4 '95	
APR 0	MY 07 92		
1985	NO 18 '92	SEP 07 1998	
AUG 3 1985	DE 15 '92	AUG 1 6 1999	
AUG 3 1985	NO 30 '93	NOV 0 9 1999	
AUG 1 1 1985		AP 7 04	
MY 16 '86	JAN 01 '95		
JUN 20 1986	JUN 28 '97	DE 1 04	
SEP 2 6 1986			
MY 07 '88	MR 07 '0		
JA 2 1 0			

ABOUT THE BOOK This timely new book addresses one of the most vital and frequently asked questions facing educators today: What implications do current brain studies have for the classroom teacher? In simple, nontechnical language the author tackles this question by

1. Briefly sketching the history of brain study

2. Presenting current concepts of brain functioning

3. Describing illustrative teaching activities (from various content areas and grade levels) keyed to brain functioning

4. Presenting a brain-compatible plan for program development

5. Outlining educational futures consistent with current trends in brain research

For those interested in the enormous educational implications of current brain research, this clearly written little primer should be must reading.

ABOUT THE AUTHOR Michael P. Grady received his doctorate in Curriculum and Instruction from Saint Louis University, where he is currently Acting Chair of the Department of Communications. The author of numerous journal articles and monographs, he co-authored EDUCATION AND THE BRAIN, a very successful monograph in Phi Delta Kappan's Fast Back Series.

0-582-28377-9